CW00688609

CURSE IN VERSE
AND
MUCH MORE WORSE

To Matthew

with thanks for your support over the years!

Love from

Trish x

by

Trish Dainton

**Grosvenor House
Publishing Limited**

All rights reserved
Copyright © Trish Dainton, 2011

Trish Dainton is hereby identified as author of this
work in accordance with Section 77 of the Copyright, Designs
and Patents Act 1988

The book cover picture is copyright to Trish Dainton

This book is published by
Grosvenor House Publishing Ltd
28-30 High Street, Guildford, Surrey, GU1 3HY.
www.grosvenorhousepublishing.co.uk

This book is sold subject to the conditions that it shall not, by way of
trade or otherwise, be lent, resold, hired out or otherwise circulated
without the author's or publisher's prior consent in any form of binding or
cover other than that in which it is published and
without a similar condition including this condition being imposed
on the subsequent purchaser.

A CIP record for this book
is available from the British Library

ISBN 978-1-908105-09-7

To my late husband Steve.

**Thank you for choosing me, and for entrusting me
to travel your journey with you.**

Stephen (Steve) Dainton 14 May 1961 – 27 January 2011

Poem for Steve

Your struggle now is over,
You fought it to the end.
I'm sorry my dear darling,
HD I could not mend.

You kept your grace and dignity,
A man so sweet and kind;
The Steve I knew and loved so much,
Was never left behind.

It tried to break your spirit,
This thing they call HD,
But never did I hear those words,
"Why did it choose me?"

And in the end, with mercy shown,
Your dignity in death.
God never let you die alone,
I witnessed your last breath.

Contents

Acknowledgements

I want to thank all the Members of the Huntington's Disease Association (HDA) Message Board for sharing with me, either directly or indirectly, their experiences through posting up messages and corresponding with me. Thank you also for your encouragement and your thoughts on my poems and observations along the way.

Thank you to Hugh Marriott and Jimmy Pollard for allowing me to write my own take on being a carer on the back of all your wisdom. Although labelled as fiction, John Harding's works also helped to broaden my understanding of the relationship between patient and carer.

I am grateful to those whose works I have also cited in the book, attributed accordingly, having searched for information on-line or in guidance books.

Finally, although this version is unauthorised by the HDA, I wanted to acknowledge their role in enabling me to write the forerunner to this book (Curse in Verse). Their help and encouragement has been invaluable, as has their care support for me and my late husband over the years.

Introduction to this book

In 2005 my husband, Steve, was diagnosed with Huntington's disease (HD). I was aware from the very beginning of our relationship that my husband had a 50% chance of inheriting HD. His father was in mid to late stages of the illness when we met and, if passed on to my husband, our children would also have a 50% chance of inheriting. Our life choices were based on the very real threat of HD.

Denial is a common thing with HD and Steve was clearly in denial, (or should that be 'unawareness?') for several years before his actual diagnosis. I guess I was as much in denial as he was. Facing up to the devastation it brings is never easy, especially when you have already watched it destroy loved ones. His father was one of eight children, with six of the children inheriting the disease from their father.

As the wife of someone who suffered from HD, and his full time carer until his death in January 2011, I have been an active Member of the Huntington's Disease Association (HDA) and its Message Board.

Curse in Verse and Much More Worse was borne out of an awareness exercise for HD and the HDA itself. The original book was entitled simply 'Curse in Verse' and contained 41 poems in all. More detail on the original concept is given in the Introduction to Section One – Mind the Awareness Gap!

The HDA currently print off and distribute Curse in Verse and have helped me in promoting it. Grateful though I am to the HDA, I since found myself working on more and more poems and wanting to spread my wings beyond the constraints of being tied to the HDA where using their resources and logo.

Many of the new poems in here, especially in the later Sections, may be viewed as provocative or even controversial in their subject matter. Being mindful of the HDA's position, I took the decision to self-publish this work which has been unauthorised.

A number of books, goods and services are mentioned by name in this book. Please note I have received no payments or inducements by any person, supplier or organisation to feature them.

This latest version containing around seventy poems, including most of the original 41, does not set out in any way to work in opposition to the HDA or its Members. I truly hope people can see I aim to compliment them in every sense of the word and, by donating all eventual profit from the sale of this book, ultimately I hope to raise funds as well as awareness.

Many of the subject matters I have covered in this book will no doubt prompt the reader to search out further information. The HDA provide a number of useful Fact Sheets which are available through their office or can be downloaded from the HDA Website **www.hda.org.uk**

At the time of writing the original book along with many of the poems for this version, Steve was in what I would term mid to late stage into progression. Sadly Steve died whilst I was working on Curse in Verse and Much More Worse. He died on January 27th 2011. It was just a few months before he would have reached the age of fifty and a few months after our twenty second wedding anniversary. The poem on the dedication page was written for his funeral.

My husband was weakened physically and mentally by the disease and, as with so many other sufferers, pneumonia took hold where his body was so weak. He was a very brave and proud man and accepted his lot with grace and dignity. After his death I decided I would continue work on this book in his memory.

It stands to reason that this book is more likely to attract those with a connection to HD. However, being the disease that it is, I'd like to think my writings can touch on any number of diseases and the role of being a carer in general.

I remember the first time I read the John Harding book 'What we did on our holiday'. The book was centrally based on a family coping with Parkinson's disease but in many ways he was describing a family which could have been living with Huntington's disease. I connected with his characters profoundly.

I'm sure that it is no accident that Hugh Marriott's book 'The Selfish Pig's Guide to Caring' was able to reach out to carers in all walks of life. I dare say Hugh's experience in caring for someone with HD played a big part in his being able to identify with all manner of frustrations and circumstances given the complexity of the disease.

A big difference between this book and those of John Harding and Hugh Marriott (apart from them being brilliant writers whereas I am an amateur with no talent that is) is their wonderful gift of mixing humour and pathos. I apologise in advance for the lack of humour portrayed in this book.

This book is made up of eight Sections. Sections one to seven contain poems grouped within a theme. I have written Introductions to the Sections and to the poems themselves. The length of the Introductions varies greatly. Some of the subject matters were simply more close to my heart resulting in it either being easier for me to elaborate on, or sometimes on the other side of the coin, too painful to.

Section eight does not contain poetry. The final section is formed out of various writing exercises I have used for therapy/fundraising/tributes. I have also included a story written by another HDA Message Board Member about her daughter who had Juvenile Huntington's Disease.

In the case of the Message Board being a direct source of work or inspiration, unless requested otherwise I have used the persons' Message Board User Name within the appropriate piece to attribute them. Permission prior to using was sought and my intention to publish the book has been well documented on the Message Board itself.

In terms of the situations within the poems themselves, any direct similarities to actual Members of the Message Board are purely coincidental. Where not arising from my own personal experience and outlined in the Introduction to the poem, the poems have been formed and inspired out of the thousands of posts I have read over the last few years covering hundreds of Members' plights. They are therefore an amalgam of stories condensed into a few short lines.

Including myself in this, it stands to reason that those who join and open their hearts on the Message Board are initially there for the same reason. They have reached the point where they are crying out for help and needing to know they are not alone. In view of this, and having subjected myself to hours and hours of pouring through posts in a bid to try capturing the essence of a particular dilemma, it's understandable my poems are more likely to be sad rather than uplifting. It also therefore follows not all cases of HD are as bleak as this book may portray, and not all elements of the disease will manifest themselves within the sufferer or those looking after them.

Because of the nature of the disease, covering physical, mental, emotional and cognitive areas of ones being, I will not have been able to represent all of the facets. It is important to state, whilst I have never set out to misrepresent HD, the context of what I have been basing my poetic creativity on will always have been swayed by my own experience of how it manifested itself in my husband and what appears to be the bleakness of the disease. Having said that... I am aware that compared to many carers my own experience has been a walk in the park.

Finally, please note, apart from personal experience in coping with being a carer for someone with HD, I have absolutely no medical training; care training; or professional background when referring to medical and professional care giving information. I simply have a questioning mind and have used reading matter and the internet to help guide me. In this respect, whatever is stated in this book is simply based on my own limited research and the views of others and is in no way provides a substitute for professional guidance.

---

* Posts submitted on the Message Board are already in the public domain. HDA or Board membership is not required to view, only to participate and submit entries.

Section 1

Mind
The
Awareness
Gap!

Please Mind the gap,
Between the platform and the train.
Please note the void,
Between awareness and the brain!

Introduction to Section 1

Mind the Awareness Gap

In June 2009, Members of the Huntington's Disease Association (HDA) Message Board were asked by one of the other Members (DH) to put their thinking caps on and give ideas on raising HD awareness. The initial thinking was to work with the HDA on a poster campaign. The posters were hoped to be seen within London through the public transport infrastructure. The aim was to coincide with HD Awareness Week 2010.

I threw in my own thoughts but it was clear with a subject like HD it was never going to be easy. Should they go for shock tactic? Should they go for softly, softly? Too much information? Too little information? Was it to inform the general public or aimed at those facing HD? Was it to raise funds? Could it do more harm than good because of the underlying fear of the public and family and friends' reactions?

I was aware of a Transport for London project called 'Poems on the Underground'. This started me thinking about the power of words in verse, and how they could be informative and emotive as well as entertaining. Also, with the use of verse, I imagined people would be more likely to read to the end of the poster. That being instead of switching off the moment they thought it was something which would not directly affect them.

I started off with a couple of poems and then felt I would just add a couple more. The next thing I knew I had seven poems. The first seven poems in this Section were those written for the initial exercise. Indeed, 'The Awareness Dream' and 'The Hope' were directed at grabbing a public response. However, by now even I could see we would need a lot of posters, or to take up the space of one of those huge posters you see facing you on the Station platform. Let's face it... it wasn't going to happen.

Having unleashed my creative juices I thought "What the heck!" Let's carry on doing my little verses anyway and see if I could try channelling this into something useful to the HDA. Even though they may be utter rubbish I could maybe get a few donations if someone felt sorry for me having wasted all my time?

In August 2009 I approached the HDA with the first set of poems in a bid to ask if there was any possibility of working on a joint project. A session at the forthcoming HDA Family Conference was covering 'interesting' ways to raise funds. I had in mind for the HDA to print up copies and pitch the work as an expressive way to raise awareness and funds.

The HDA didn't laugh and throw the idea straight back at me, although they may be regretting that now. Instead they suggested we try it out for size at the World Congress in Vancouver. No pressure..!

Poems eight to twelve do not feature in the original book. I have written and added them subsequently as I wanted to convey things are moving forward in the awareness stakes. There is still a long way to go however.

The Test

Introduction

Every child born to a person with HD, regardless of gender, has a 50 percent chance of inheriting the faulty gene.

A test is available to determine whether or not a person has inherited it. If tested as 'positive' the person knows they are likely to go on to develop the illness at some point in their lives. In the UK the minimum age for a person requesting the 'Predictive Test' is currently eighteen.

With no cure as yet for what is a devastating condition, whether to take the test or not is a very personal and difficult decision to make especially when the odds are as high as 50/50.

Sat in hospital waiting room,
He sits with tissue ready.
The call comes out to enter room,
He stands, his legs unsteady.

He steps inside, he's offered seat;
The Doctor meets his eye.
He feels himself start to go numb,
Determined not to cry.

The words come from the Doctor's mouth,
He doesn't want to hear.
Among the words one word stands out,
"It's **positive** I fear."

The Doctor's arm around him now,
He leads him from the room.
He knows there is no cure as yet,
He feels he faces doom.

The Sufferer

Introduction

This poem tries to convey how society sometimes judges and poorly treats HD sufferers. There are many different ways in which a person with HD may be misjudged by society but I have used the assumption of being drunk here.

My poor husband experienced a lot of ignorant looks of disdain, and cruel comments, but apart from wearing a tee-shirt emblazoned with something like 'I am not drunk, I have HD!' what can you do? Even then the tee shirt would have to explain what HD is on the back.

Sadly there are occasions where people with HD are assumed by the public to be drunk to the extent of calling the police where they have fallen, or their behaviour leads people to assume police intervention is required.

She sits in chair while people stare,
Her body thin and weak.
She cannot stand, control her hand,
She slurs when trying to speak.

A passing stranger gives a look,
As if to say, 'You're drunk!'
A common thing, to look at her,
And think 'how low she's sunk!'

If only they knew half the truth,
Perhaps their scorn would stop.
Her genes the blame for all her shame,
She hasn't touched a drop.

And yet the filthy looks go on,
And ignorance is rife.
She knows that things will get worse still,
She knows this is her life.

The Generations

Introduction

Because HD does not normally skip generations, if a child becomes symptomatic (Juvenile HD - JHD) it will be a case of the child having inherited it directly from the affected parent. It therefore suggests the parent's fate too if they were not already tested or symptomatic.

It is more likely than not that the parent will have become symptomatic and have been diagnosed as HD positive before their child reaches their own symptoms. However, unless the parent does not share the home, they will still sadly have to witness HD together in the cruellest of ways.

He stands above his restless child,
Her body thrashing out.
She's tired and thin, just bone and skin,
He hears her scream and shout.

His heart is breaking every time,
He goes into her room.
What should have been a happy time,
Has been replaced with gloom.

Just how much time do they still have?
Too little time he's sure.
He knows their fate because of this,
He's seen it once before.

The gene is passing down the line,
He since has come to learn.
He watched his dad die, now his child,
And next will be his turn.

The Carer

Introduction

HD manifests itself in physical and mental deterioration over a number of years. Imagine having to look after someone with Parkinson's; Motor Neurone and Alzheimer's among other types of illness rolled into one.

The strains of looking after someone who is so dependant takes its toll on the Carer to the point of often having to let them go for their own and the patient's safety. Sometimes the guilt is the hardest part.

The above wording was used for the Introduction to this poem in the original Curse in Verse. When writing it I was terrified things might develop to the point where I would have to put my husband in a nursing home. Keeping him at home was always down to his condition not worsening beyond what I could cope with mentally or physically. It would only have taken an accident on the part of either and I am sure the decision would have been taken away from me.

In twenty four years of knowing him, and all through his HD, my husband was hospitalised on just two occasions. He had a chest infection which he caught from a relative passing onto him the Norovirus, and at one point we thought he had suffered a stroke. In each case he was hospitalised for one night only. Having refused to leave his side I dare say part of releasing him early was down to wanting to get me out of the hospital too!

Did I do him any favours? I'd like to think so as he always seemed grateful to me for keeping him at home. I will never know if he might have been better off in a Care Home with professional full-time care. There were many times I did wonder...

I was never under the same sort of pressure as many carers and I hated using the word 'guilt' in my original introduction. No one should feel any sense of guilt when faced with having to make such hard choices, or having choices forced upon them, under such difficult circumstances.

Only yesterday it seems,
They started married life.
So full of love and hopes and dreams,
The new husband and wife.

His soul mate once so spirited,
Has now become a shell.
The empty eyes stare back at him,
It feels like living hell.

Each day he lives in turmoil.
Why is life so unfair?
Does she even know my name?
Does she even care?

A nursing home is not far off.
If not, he fears he'll drown!
"In sickness and in health" they vowed,
He feels he's let her down.

The Baby

Introduction

This poem reflects on the sadness of losing one's faculties as the illness progresses. At the time of writing this – November 2009 - my husband was seven months into wearing incontinence pants and pads ('inco pants' as termed here).

We were waiting on an appointment to discuss insertion into his stomach of a Percutaneous Endoscopic Gastroscopy (PEG) tube to help try bypassing the swallowing issues that can come with HD. In the end my husband chose not to have a PEG fitted.

He lays there gently in her womb,
A child in purest state.
Yet deep inside there lies a fault,
A gene to mar his fate.

His body feeding through a cord,
At birth cord cut, no pain.
Now 50 years from being born,
The cord attached again.

The babe, as was, lies in his bed,
The bar sides raised like cot.
The inco pants, where nappies once,
Control again forgot.

He lies there wriggling like a baby,
PEG tube in, so sore.
The only way of feeding now,
A babe in womb once more.

The Awareness Dream

Introduction

In this poem, apart from wanting to note society's general ignorance around the illness, I wanted to highlight even those with HD in their families can try to ignore it exists or acknowledge the high risk of inheriting.

Denial is actually a big part of living with HD and there is a big problem with people not being told of the risks of passing on HD to their children, thereby not being given the opportunity to make life decisions before it is too late.

As I detailed in the Introduction to this Section, this poem was one written for an exercise in public awareness. Cancer used to be a dirty word years ago but public awareness and advancement in treatments now mean it is not as hidden as it once was. Let's hope that one day families of those with HD will be able to be more open. There may not be a cure as I write but, knowledge can give empowerment at least.

The words on paper can't convey,
The sadness felt inside,
That whilst awareness is the key,
So many want to hide.

The shame felt by those suffering;
The name that is unspoken.
Society has made them scared,
Their minds and spirit broken.

Yet one day maybe strangers,
Will take the time of day,
To read the poems set in print,
As they go on their way.

And some will find out more and more,
To understand the plight,
Of those who suffer Huntington's,
An illness they can't fight.

The Hope

Introduction

Here I have tried to remember those affected by HD must never give up hope that a cure, or at least better treatment, may be just around the corner. There is a lot of hope!

Organisations like the CHDI Foundation (informally known as the Cure Huntington's disease initiative) are working flat out to find a cure or better treatment for HD. CHDI is a private, not-for-profit, research organisation dedicated purely to HD. The CHDI work with an international network of scientists who are working together towards discovering drugs that slow the progression or delay the onset of HD.
www.highqfoundation.org

Until such time when scientists are in a position to make their work transfer to patients and potential patients, the HDA and fellow organisations will be there to hold peoples' hands.

She writes the poems, one by one,
And reads them back at length.
They paint a picture hard to bear,
It's taken all her strength.

And yet she feels the picture's wrong,
It's lacking, incomplete.
It's missing sense of hope and help,
It's lost in its defeat.

The picture does look bleak it's true,
But who is there to say,
With public's help and knowledge found,
A cure's not on its way?

So if you've taken time to read,
And feel moved by her verse.
Please think of those with Huntington's,
And help us cure this curse.

The Patrons

Introduction

The Huntington's Disease Association was founded in 1971 as a self help group with 76 members. It was then known as the Association to Combat Huntington's Chorea. At that time families lived in complete isolation, unaware of the extent of the disease in the community and stigmatised by its hereditary nature.

In 1997 The Countess of Harewood kindly gave her patronage to the Association. The Countess came into contact with the HDA through her daughter-in-law who was 'at risk'. Fortunately her daughter-in-law tested negative. To have Royal Patronage became a tremendous boost to the plight of those with HD and their families and we owe a huge debt of gratitude to the Countess.

In 2009 the HDA was able to announce another boost to raising the profile of HD by adding Tony Hadley of Spandau Ballet fame, and Shane Richie of Eastenders fame, as Patrons.

Tony's connection with HD is cited as having seen a relative die from HD and having first-hand knowledge of the disease.

Shane is cited as becoming involved where he came to learn about the disease when doing research for a storyline in Eastenders. His research made him come to realise what a "tough time families of people with Huntington's disease have".

Again, we are truly indebted to Tony and Shane for becoming HDA Patrons.

From single voice, a cry for help, someone lends a hand,
Before too long another reaches out to help them stand.
Once standing up on sinking sand they ask for solid ground,
To stop them sinking down again they need a platform sound.

The lucky ones find platform comes, from those who want to share,
Their luck in life when looking at the helpless standing there.
Foundations now begin to form, upon which strong things grow,
And others start to notice them, where Patronage will show.

With the Patrons comes awareness, with them comes attention,
A worthy cause once never heard will now receive a mention.
The media so fickle will begin to look and see,
If they think there is a Royal link or spot 'celebrity'

And the single voice that cried for help is stood on shoulders high,
No longer going under while their hands reach for the sky.
The busy Patrons give their time, as much as they can spare,
Their names alone are priceless gifts to show how much they care.

The Prevalence

Introduction

On June 30th 2010 The Lancet published an article by Sir Michael Rawlins, Chairman of the National Institute of Health and Clinical Excellence (NICE). The article, entitled 'Huntington's disease out of the closet?' underlined the need to pin down more data on the real prevalence of HD.

As a lay person reading the article, Sir Michael raises questions about the possible underestimation in the prevalence of HD. A prevalence estimate of 12.4 per 100,000 of the population of England and Wales was given as a minimum, based on the HDA having 6,702 diagnosed cases of HD on their books at the time of calculating.

Sir Michael highlights gaps in the capture of numbers where the HDA could not be expected to know of all cases in England and Wales. The figures known could only formally be based on referrals from health practitioners. The stigma surrounding the disease means many people do not seek diagnosis either through fear of the outcome or through ignorance of the disease being in the family and/or its inheritance risk.

The article also spoke of the need to better know the numbers in order to plan for the future. Finance and resources need to be made available to cope with the complex needs of HD. Not just in terms of the symptomatic patient but those at risk and going through the testing stages.

Alongside the above, Sir Michael raises the need to tackle the disease head on by increasing research resources. By investing more in research to delay or ultimately stop progression, which needs far more concentration on pre-symptomatic patients, the drain on resources and strain on families will be less in the future.

Just out of interest, I posted up on the HDA Message Board a question.

I asked Members to add stories of instances where they had randomly come across others affected by HD. Bearing in mind how rare this disease is said to be...

Within a short time a number of Members came along with stories of coming across HD by chance. This included one lady whose first cousin met and married a man with HD just as she had done so. However, the husbands were from different towns and totally unrelated. Then there was her neighbour who had worked with a man who had HD, and then there was a young man attending the same school as her grandchild who also had HD in the family.

For my own part, my husband's friend at school married a woman with HD in her family; my brother in law's ex girlfriend's adopted father had HD; a friend of mine only recently discovered a HD link to foster children he grew up with, and our local jeweller's father-in-law had HD. I found that out when having my husband's wedding ring changed where his weight had plummeted and mentioned HD was why there would be a hand tremor.

I do accept if someone is looking for something then they are much more likely to find it, but surely the odds of coming across totally unrelated cases of HD shouldn't be that high if it is meant to be that rare?

"He fell again", says the wife on the phone,
As she chatters with her husband's brother.
"Tell him to take it with water next time,
He's beginning to sound like our mother".

The father had walked out on mother years back;
The boys had blamed that on her drinking.
What they couldn't have known was depression and booze,
Was just part of her balance and thinking.

When seeing the Doctor several weeks on,
He's asked if there's anything known,
Of similar traits in the family tree,
Where example of things can be shown?

"None at all" says the husband,
Believing he's first to have something they cannot explain,
Not aware of the gene that was passed down the line,
As the doctor asks questions in vain.

Unbeknown to the boys in a town far away,
Their step-sister had hidden the news,
She'd worked out for herself that their mother was ill,
But was too scared to tell them her views.

Having married a man who had worked in a place,
Where a colleague with HD had been,
They discussed the disease, and with unnerving ease,
She identified symptoms she'd seen.

22

With awareness she'd found that HD was renowned,
To have stigma and keep itself 'hid',
And with step-brother's children to add to dilemma,
She opted to keep on a lid.

So for several years more the oblivious sibling,
Was on his GP's door still knocking,
With tests and prescriptions signed off all the while,
And their NHS costs which were shocking!

When finally everything else is ruled out,
And Huntington's comes in to play,
The step-sister mentions she'd known all along,
But was worried about what to say.

The budget forecasts are due in next month;
He puts '1' in the 'Cases – HD',
But he knows with the mother, and children and brother,
The Doctor could count at least three!

The HD APPG

Introduction

In 'The Prevalence' I wrote about a milestone article for HD published in The Lancet on June 30th 2010. The timing of that article was to coincide with another milestone event held that day. The launch of the 'All Party Parliamentary Group [APPG] on Huntington's Disease'.

As the name suggests, All Party groups are formed in Parliament by MPs and peers who come from both Houses and various political parties. They are not controlled by the party whips. This allows to a higher degree non-partial discussion and representation for causes in their own right. It also helps ensure the issues facing those represented are less likely to be lost sight of when governments debate policies which will affect the causes covered by APPGs.

The APPG on Huntington's' aim is stated to be:

'To raise the public profile of Huntington's Disease and give a voice in Parliament to those suffering from the disease as well as their families and carers.'

The importance of the APPG and the launch event, which was attended by hundreds of sufferers and supporters, was acknowledged in the House of Commons. Printed below is an excerpt from Hansard - the printed transcript of Parliamentary business. The excerpt is from the proceedings of 1st July 2010.

'Mr Mark Williams (Ceredigion) (LD): *The Deputy Leader of the House [Mr David Heath CBE MP] is aware of the impressive lobby of this place yesterday by the Huntington's Disease Association. Will he give us time for a debate to consider the challenges facing the 6,700 people diagnosed with Huntington's disease, particularly those to do with accessing insurance and the adequacy of research into a hitherto incurable disease?*

Mr Heath: *I am grateful to my hon. Friend for that question. I, too, yesterday met constituents who either had Huntington's disease or who were caring for people with Huntington's disease. It brought home to all Members of the House who had contact with those people how difficult the disease is to manage. It is a degenerative disease with a genetic component that imposes a great deal of stress both on those who contract it and those who care for them. I know that* *there are clear issues about future research and the sort of support that can be given at the point of diagnosis and the point of management in GP practices and elsewhere in order to help. I understand that an all-party parliamentary group on Huntington's disease has been established and that is a welcome step forward. I cannot promise my hon. Friend a debate in the next two weeks, I am afraid, but he might care to apply for an Adjournment debate or a Westminster Hall debate on this important subject.'*

The following is by way of a Roll Call for those who helped form the APPG and made the launce event such a success. There were no doubt others I have missed here for which I do apologise.

Many thanks must be extended to:

Sir Michael Rawlins, whose idea it was to create an APPG and for adding weight behind what many of us have suspected all along. HD is far wider spread than people like to admit.

Charles Sabine, BBC and NBC war correspondent who put so much energy into the launch and who is also fighting and corresponding on his own personal war (Charles is HD Positive).

Cath Stanley and the HDA team and Members including Matt Ellison who made the launch event so well orchestrated, attended, and powerful.

Those who gave financial support; media support; and support in kind including Martyn Lewis and family; Adrian Flook (M Communications), Jayne Innes, Quintin Clover, The Bickerdike family, Don and Shirley Moody, Jane Cavangh, Nick Doff, NICE TV, and Doctor and Mrs AR Gillespie.

The attending HD Patrons Tony Hadley and Sarah Winkless.

The supportive and attending eminent names in the fields of HD science and research including Sarah Tabrizi, Ed Wild and Alice and Nancy Wexler. The Wexler family have been instrumental in the identification of the gene that causes Huntington's which is paramount in finding a cure.

The volunteers from Track, EHDN and all the HDA regions.

The hundreds of families and supporters who attended the event launch.

Last but not least, thanks must be extended to the 37 or so Members of the House of Commons and Lords who stood up to be counted and formed the APPG.

Democracy, apparently, is there for one and all,
But look at any Hansards and the argument will stall.
It's clear to see that policy may form from strong debate,
But what if Party ignorance wrongly seals a fate?

OK there is the process where you write to your MP,
And try to get across your case amongst all those they see.
Fighting for attention, and hoping they will care,
You're writing as an advocate about things so unfair!

But now there is some hope out there for those who have HD,
A Group's been formed on Huntington's, a new A.P.P.G.
Where once HD was swept aside, because of Party choice,
A new All Party Group now stands, to give us all a voice!

Section 2

The
Appliance
Of
Science

I realise I may not have,
A medical degree;
But who's to say your trainings',
Not distorting what you see?

Introduction to Section 2

The Appliance of Science

The poems within this Section have been grouped to broadly cover some of the research and medical aspects of being a patient and carer as I, and others, have perceived them. As previously stated I have no medical background or expertise other than what I have learnt and researched over the course of looking after my husband and writing my poems.

The final poem in this Section 'The Gay' could have slotted into any number of the other Sections. I have added it in here as it highlights one of the areas where misdiagnosis may be made leading to all manner of issues. The added danger of the medical profession acting in a less than objective fashion worried me.

The point above is borne out again in Section 8 'Rikki's Story' where the age of the person led to delay in diagnosis. In Rikki's case there was reluctance on the part of the medical professional to consider HD. It therefore needs to be reiterated that the disease shows no prejudice and affects all genders; sexual orientations; races; ages; life styles etc etc.

Misdiagnosis can work both ways of course. There is always a danger of reading HD into symptoms where it could be something different affecting the person. For example 'Picks disease' or 'neuroacanthocytosis'. At least with HD the gene test can rule out the disease as much as rule it in thus allowing for further investigation.

It is clear that the future of HD lies in the hands of scientific researchers. However, it is also clear that until more answers and treatments come forward the welfare of the patients lies in the hands of carers. It's not the sort of illness you can simply self medicate to control.

I do feel I may be taking out my anger at HD on the very people who are doing their best to help by being so negative in my poems at times. Resources are such that they are working under extreme difficulty. By default we remember and hear about the bad more than the good experiences. That said... I feel it would be just as wrong of me not to pick up on some of the areas of concern having come out of my own experiences and those of others.

On the whole, it is fair to say my husband received a very high standard of care from the medical teams we came across and I have a lot of admiration for those involved. That is not to say I blindly trusted everyone as having more knowledge than me. I knew my husband better than anyone.

My own personality is such that to be able to be a good carer and advocate for my husband I felt I needed to learn about the disease and demonstrate a basic understanding and respect for it. Whether that approach was a healthy one to take, or the right for everyone, it is not for me to say. I know I just felt a lot better having some sort of empowerment by way of knowledge.

The HD+ Optimist

Introduction

This poem was written for a friend of mine who tested positive for the gene. It never fails to amaze me how some of the people in HD circles that I have come across, who know they have the gene, remain so positive about life.

My friend is doing everything he can to continue life as normal as possible. Not in a denial fashion but not letting the disease eat away at him before it has even started to take hold. Part of his control is being proactive instead of reactive and taking steps to keep as healthy as possible, as happy as possible, and be on medical and research programmes so that he is in the right place at the right time when the breakthroughs come.

I refer to 'CAG' in this poem. The CAG count of a person tested is the indicator of whether or not they are likely to develop HD. An extract from the HDA's Fact Sheet on Predictive Testing for HD is given below:

The Huntington's Gene

Genes are made up of DNA (deoxyribonucleic acid). DNA itself is made up of four chemicals which are known by letters of the alphabet:
*   C Cytosine A Adenine G Guanine T Thymine*

One section of the Huntington's gene contains three of these chemicals – CAG – repeated a number of times. In the faulty gene these three chemicals are repeated many times, like a 'molecular stutter'.

Four types of results are recognised: Under 27 repeats is unequivocally normal. Between 27-35 repeats is normal but there is a small chance that the repeat may increase in future generations. Between 36-39 repeats the result is abnormal but there is a chance the person may be affected very late in life or even not at all. Over 40 repeats is unequivocally abnormal.

Though the test can tell whether you carry the Huntington's disease mutation, it cannot tell you when the disease itself will start to develop.

So he's just had his result from the doctor,
And the news wasn't good to hear.
His CAG showed that he, is a HD to be,
But it didn't fill him with great fear.

You see he's done all his research a plenty,
And he's not the type just to give in.
He's looked on the 'Net', and whilst nothings' there yet,
He knows this is something he'll win!

There's a whole world out there doing research,
And the signs look like one day they'll find,
A cure for the neuro disorders,
It's simply a matter of time.

So he'll do what he needs to do right now,
To keep himself fit and prepared,
Because he and those 'HD Ready',
Are surely to have their lives spared!

The Fighter

Introduction

This poem tries to reflect how those with HD, at risk pre-symptomatic or symptomatic, may look to alternative medicine such as supplements to help stave off the illness. It touches on the reluctance of some of the medical profession to accept their ways aren't the only way and how I feel, if it was they who had HD, they too would go to any lengths.

It is worth adding here that if embarking upon taking supplements the fact that such substances may have a beneficial effect also means they may have an adverse effect. The poem below raises a reluctance by some of the medical profession (not all I hasten to add) to embrace alternative medicine. That aside... It is always advisable to consult with your GP before self administering.

Where I decided to try my husband on creatine I informed his doctor and neurologist. I was able to reassure them that I had taken steps to ensure the supply was from a reputable company who sold pharmaceutical grade creatine. I was also able to display I was aware of the need for monitoring levels of fluid intake.

To be safe however, we arranged regular blood checks given the potential for damage to the liver and kidneys. Being aware of the supplements which included creatine, cod liver oil with Omega3 and Vitamin C with Zinc, the physicians were also able to factor this in when prescribing drugs lest there be a reaction.

I have stressed the above points as in another poem 'The Cocktail' I highlight the dangers of mixing medicines without taking account of interaction with other meds. It stands to reason therefore that supplements and other non-prescribed factors may also play their part if things go wrong.

When things look bleak, I must believe,
I'm cleverer, than this disease.
Surely a way, to keep at bay,
And bring this cruel thing, to its' knees?

I find each day, another way,
To counter weapons, that it throws.
Research I've done, second to none,
The hours spent, the strain, it shows.

33

And all the money; spend obscene,
Blueberries, fish oils, creatine.
He looks at me, like I'm a fool,
This Doctor, years from Medic School.

The notes are scribbled, on my file.
That look he gives me, all the while.
He thinks I'm stupid, should feel shame,
YOU live with this, YOU'D do the same!

The Guinea Pig

Introduction

Here I try to express the sheer desperation of those wanting to be part of trials in the hope they will be part of a cure. It cannot be understated how vital it is to have people sign up for participation in studies and research. It not only makes sense in terms of the bigger picture, but those taking part at an early stage in their diagnosis (if not before) are in a better position to benefit more quickly when the time comes.

There are a number of research projects taking place at any one time. One example is TRACK-HD:

'As a comprehensive study of pre-manifest and early HD, TRACK-HD aims to measure the sensitivity of individual and combined assessment tools to detect subtle changes in disease progression. The ultimate goal is to establish what combination of measures is the most sensitive for detecting change over the natural course of HD. This would lay the foundations to develop the much needed methodology to undertake future clinical trials of disease-modifying agents in HD.'

Source: www.track-hd.net

He's signed up all the paperwork,
And looked up all the rest.
He's hoping they will choose his name,
To be part of this test.

A 'Wonder drug' he's heard it called,
He knows from reading text;
The drug it works for Alzheimer's,
And HD will be next.

He's conscious of the risks involved,
He knows it may go wrong;
But what if it gives him more time?
The argument is strong.

And so he waits with baited breath,
His last hope this is true.
He grabs the phone on second ring,
To hear that he got through.

The Lab Rat

Introduction

I was asked to take the following poem out of my original Curse in Verse book. I could see there was merit in doing so given the sensitivity of the subject matter. I complied but always felt uncomfortable with it as I felt I was letting the poor creatures down. I'm not saying I condone testing on animals, in fact I'd rather more **consenting** human testing be used but recognise the minefield of ethics.

Whatever your own personal feelings about laboratory testing on animals the fact remains that, as I type this book, all over the world animals are being used for experimentation. Not just for HD but to help create treatments and cures for all human and animal diseases known to mankind.

In view of the above I wanted to recognise the plight of laboratory animals. Many animals are used from mice to sheep and their efforts deserved to be recognised as much as anyone else.

The creature lays there in its cage,
The wires to its head.
It's been injected for so long,
It really should be dead.

And yet its tiny heart beats strong,
Its body fighting back.
It has no sense of what it has,
Or how the genes attack.

The next day when the human comes,
She feeds him feeling numb.
She cannot dare to even care,
The animal is 'dumb'.

But everyone with HD knows,
That 'dumb' is not the score.
They owe a debt of gratitude,
To him and thousands more!

The Researcher

Introduction

This poem touches on the hope that a cure is out there. But what about those who say no one would want to research into cures for HD anyway with it being an 'orphan' disease (a condition so rare it doesn't make it financially viable for the drug industries to spend resources on)? I was one of those sceptical people but several months after writing my poem I read some encouraging news.

'HDBuzz' an on-line HD research news magazine, written by scientists in plain language, featured an article in March 2011. It was an interview with the Global Head for Neuroscience at Novartis. The article was encouraging in that it wrote:

'We started by asking Bilbe why Novartis got into HD research when, financially, it might seem more sensible to work on more common brain diseases. Degenerative brain diseases like HD and Alzheimer's, he answered, are all "chronic, they're slow, they're really tough", which makes them expensive to study and difficult to treat. In addition, most such diseases strike at random: "We don't really know who are the patients we're going to treat" so developing drugs to prevent them is even harder. After a long time trying, the pharmaceutical industry has found working with degenerative brain diseases very frustrating, with millions of affected people and very few successes.

HD is different, says Bilbe. Because we know exactly what genetic mutation causes HD, "we believe we can beat the odds. We know who the patients are, and that makes the whole process of drug discovery and knowing how to test your drug, and which patients it should work in, a lot more predictable."

Source: Interview with Graeme Bilbe, Global Head for Neuroscience at Novartis, written by Dr Ed Wild. www.HDBuzz.net

Sounds encouraging but let's just hope that when the day comes the inequality of a postcode lottery on healthcare, as seen with drugs for other illnesses such as cancer, doesn't mean treatment will be withheld due to inadequate funds and resources.

He's spent the last 5 years or more,
Employee of a group,
Who's paid to spook upon drug firms,
Just looking for a scoop.

There's money to be made here,
The next big thing is due.
A cure for cancer, MS, AIDS,
Common colds and flu.

He sits among the files piled deep,
As far as eyes can see.
He holds a file and starts to weep,
The title is HD.

He's never told his ruthless boss,
That money's not his lure.
His wife is HD Positive,
And now they've found a cure!

The Cocktail

Introduction

I have taken the inspiration for this poem from anecdotal evidence. It's worrying that in some cases the medical profession may prescribe drugs for symptoms not fully taking into account the adverse effects when combining drugs for a mind and body so fragile. The damage can be irreversible. Tetra B = Tetrabenazine.

Where taking supplements (see 'The Fighter') it is imperative that this is mentioned so that the system does not have any other forms of substance in it which may adversely add to the mix.

You've got HD, here's Tetra B,
A common pill to take.
There may be lots of side effects,
But least it stops the shake.

You've got HD, now let me see,
You're feeling so depressed.
Take this one... Citalopram,
You're bound to feel less stressed.

You've got HD, how can this be?
You lie most nights awake?
Here's Zopiclone to add to mix,
A better sleep to make.

You've got HD, Oh goodness me!
You're getting paranoia.
Here's Clozapine to take as well,
The 'voices' won't annoy ya.

You've got HD, Oh silly me!
Some drugs aren't meant together.
I'm sorry dear, too late I fear,
They may affect forever!

The Videofluoroscopy

Introduction

Swallowing difficulties (Dysphagia) and/or food and liquids travelling into the lungs (Aspiration) can be a common problem for patients with HD. Choking, for example, is not only distressing for the patient and those witnessing, it can lead to malnutrition and chest infections. Pneumonia, in particular in the late stage of HD, can be fatal. Speech and Language Therapy and Dietetic assistance will be invaluable to help control the problems. Where available, patients may also be offered a Videofluoroscopy.

The Videofluoroscopy takes place in the X-ray department of a hospital and the process involves X-Raying the head and neck area whilst foodstuffs and liquids are swallowed. Barium solution helps to trace the path of the swallowed substance. This helps to show up any signs of the substance bypassing the oesophagus flap and entering into the lungs instead of passing through to the stomach.

I wrote this poem quite some time before my husband died. He had two videoflouroscopy sessions with several months gap in between. As it turned out, pneumonia was given as the actual cause of his death.

I can't be sure if pneumonia was from a viral infection or if, having opted not to have a PEG fitted, his food or drink caused the final outcome. I will never know.

The coughing, the choking, the sharp gulps of air,
Another stage closer, the signs are all there.
Where once it was guess work to know how far gone,
Machines take an X-Ray to see damage done.

He cuts a frail figure whilst sat in his chair,
Alone and quite frightened, and yet I'm still there.
They hand him some water, his hands drop the cup,
My instincts resisted to wipe the mess up.

Changed thickness of drinks now, and food coated white,
The barium powder to help X-rays' sight.
I'm sat behind shield now, his skull on the screen,
My husband the skeleton now can be seen.

The Therapist commentates, doing her best,
It's clear that the food's re-directing to chest.
It won't be too long before risk of infection,
His food now a killer, through its misdirection.

The Terminology

Introduction

This poem is about the use of medical terms when referring to symptoms of the disease.

Shortly after my husband was diagnosed we were sent a copy of a letter to his doctor which was written by his Neurologist. It contained the word 'anhedonia'. I had to look the word up and it made sad reading as it brought it home to me that, whilst my husband was still showing signs of recognising 'pleasure', it could be that he would lose even that most basic form of human awareness.

Because of the complexity of the disease the chances are that many will come across words used in the description of symptoms that are not easily recognised. The majority of the terms given below were used in connection with my husband. I personally found it useful to look into the meanings of the words to try helping me get a handle on where those making assumptions about my husband were coming from.

"It's all Greek to me!" Is the phrase in my head,
As the words on the paper begin to be read.
Is it Greek, is it Latin? I haven't a clue,
But it sounds quite impressive how they describe you.

So I turn on computer and search on a word,
Oh why is the spelling of these so absurd?
And then one by one, as their meanings unfold,
It's no wonder they use them, the sadness they hold.

'Aspiration' tells me though happy you're fed,
The nutrition is aiming for your lungs instead.
'Dysphagia' tells me the food that I give,
Is making you choke more than helping you live.

'Dysarthria' tells me your mouth will not say,
What you want me to do, do you want it this way?
'Bruxism' tells me your teeth will grind more,
And whilst you do not notice, my nerves can't ignore.

'Ataxia' tells me your order is altered,
Explaining the speech and the steps that are faltered.
'Dystonia' tells I straighten in vain,
The stiff limbs contorting, contracting again.

'Alexithymia' tells me your feelings are dead,
Or you cannot express them as words can't be said.
'Anhedonia' tells me you cannot feel pleasure,
Devoid of the feelings you once used to treasure.

'Myoclonus' tells me the thrashing in bed,
And the knee in my back, and the punch in the head,
It's not that you mean it, it's not aimed at me,
There's a name for this symptom within your HD.

➢ **Alexithymia** *n.* a lack of ability to understand and communicate one's own emotions and moods. It is common in depression and can cause significant relationship difficulties during the person's illness. Source A

➢ **Anhedonia** *n.* a reduction in or the total loss of the feeling of pleasure in acts that normally give pleasure. Source A

➢ **Aspiration** *n.* the taking of foreign matter into the lungs with the respiratory current. Source B

➢ **Ataxia** *n.* an inability to coordinate voluntary muscular movements that is symptomatic of some central nervous system disorders and injuries and not due to muscle weakness. Source B

➢ **Bruxism** *n.* the habit of unconsciously gritting or grinding the teeth especially in situations of stress or during sleep. Source B

➢ **Dysarthria** *n.* difficulty in articulating words due to disease of the central nervous system. Source B

➢ **Dystonia** *n.* muscle dysfunction characterised by spasms or abnormal muscle contractions. Source A

➢ **Dysphagia** *n.* Difficulty in swallowing. Source B

➢ **Myoclonus** *n.* Irregular involuntary contraction of a muscle usually resulting from functional disorder of controlling motor neurons. Source B

Source 'A' - Oxford Concise Medical Dictionary

Source 'B' - Merriam-Webster on-line m-w.com

The Name Game

Introduction

For some time now the disease named by George Huntington has been known as 'Huntington's disease' or 'HD'. It was originally known as 'Huntington's Chorea' or 'HC' due to the noticeable involuntary movements of the people affected. The term chorea derives from the Greek word for dance 'choreia'.

As more information became known about Huntington's, and it became clear the motor/movement characteristics were just a part of the illness; and also that not all patients actually overtly displayed involuntary body movement, the term chorea was replaced by 'disease'. Many people, myself included, are unhappy with HD still being referred to by its old name. This is particularly worrying where members of the medical profession are involved.

Many of us feel compelled to point out to professionals at every opportunity the 'disease' element being important in particular where cognitive, emotional and reasoned thinking is compromised more than physical movement. To label such a complex disease as simply chorea suggests an ignorance of its true nature.

Sadly when my husband died, 'huntingtons [sic] chorea' was stated on his death certificate.

I don't have "HC", I have "HD",
I snap at the doctor in front of me.
If he mentions "chorea" just once more,
I'm in danger of kicking him out of the door!

"Chorea" may be what you heard at med school,
But by using it now you just sound like a fool.
It's been several years now it's been called 'disease',
So go back to your books and research this thing please.

Yes there may be link to 'chorea' or 'dance',
Where in olden days doctors just gave us one glance,
But in case you've not noticed it alters my mind,
And the movement's the least of my worries you'll find.

Please show me respect, and use the right name,
The 'disease' terms' important, it's not a word game.
It's used to ensure it reflects what is true,
That this thing is so complex one symptom won't do!

The Gay

Introduction

Some of the symptoms of HIV/AIDS include weight loss; lack of energy; short term memory loss; seizures and lack of coordination and confusion. They happen to be similar to the symptoms of HD.

I've heard of at least one gay couple where one of the partners started to show symptoms of HD but he wasn't aware of his family history.

Despite both parties knowing HIV was unlikely in themselves, the general assumption was HIV and they were encouraged to get tested for it. As you can imagine, before HD was finally diagnosed, there had been a whole layer of issues to be dealt with by them both.

This poem also notes HD affects people regardless of their gender, age, race or sexual orientation.

The change in attitude is clear,
And whilst it has been slow,
No longer sneers and shouts of "Queers",
But still a way to go.

Acceptance in society,
Has been a welcome side.
Now holding hands, joint wedding bands,
Their love no need to hide.

The gene it has no prejudice,
It's always been that way.
Girl or boy, black or white,
No matter, straight or gay.

There is one sad side of it though,
The side of H.I.V.
When public just assumes the case,
Though it could be HD!

Section 3

Before
The
Storm

There's one thing in being told,
A storm is on its way;
It's another when tsunami strikes,
And it's around to stay!

Introduction to Section 3

Before the Storm

The 'Storm' is what I have named the realisation of HD and what it means.

Having lived through HD with my husband, there are many things I regret we didn't look into before the disease took hold. Part of it was down to ignorance of the disease; part of it was down to the disease affecting everyone differently to a higher or lesser degree and not knowing what to plan for; part of it was down to lack of information being out there in the first place (one of the reasons I wanted to share my views and experiences); and part of it being good old fashioned denial!

This Section tries to convey some of the angles on preparation for what lies ahead and some of the frustrating elements of denial. I have ended it with 'The Bucket' list as there is always room to turn a bad situation into a good one however hard that may be to believe. I am sure I am not the only one who thinks of the "irony" when people say they have a "positive" result for HD hence using the words good and bad.

The Owl and the Ostrich

Introduction

I can't be certain but I believe the use of Owls and Ostriches, in relation to HD, originated from a speech given by Charles Sabine. Charles has been active in campaigning for HD awareness and more research towards a cure where his family, and sadly he himself, have been directly affected.

Here is my interpretation of what I think the terms mean.

The terms relate to those HD positive; negative; at risk; and even those around them such as carers, friends and colleagues.

The Owls are people who feel their best defence is to learn everything they can about the disease and, in a way, hit it straight on armed with knowledge. Thereby doing everything possible to prevent onset, or to be able to care for/relate to someone affected.

The Ostriches have a coping mechanism where they do their best to stave off what could be the inevitable by distancing themselves from it. They try to avoid facing it as far as possible, much like an ostrich with its head in the sand.

To be fair to those in denial, and who can blame them after all, I have also covered in my poems 'The Unawareness'. Here the person is said to be in unintentional denial. Not only are they totally unaware of what is happening to them, but also unable to see and accept what others can see. In essence we need to think more about whether someone has actual control over their actions in the first place before we can accuse them of doing something.

It's not for me to say which is the right approach or the wrong one. Everyone copes differently as best they can. I have tended to be an owl whereas my husband was an ostrich in the context of this poem. He was happy in his own little world and I was, or should I say still am, happy in mine.

Devouring the words in front of her,
The books piled upon the table,
She looks at all the reference tools,
Her knowledge to enable.

She feels that if she understands,
The thing they call HD,
She's better armed to win the fight,
Against her enemy.

Yet in another room he lies,
Her brother on his bed,
He's just as likely to succumb,
But doesn't fill his head.

He feels his way is just as good,
Avoiding all the stress,
His 'ignorance is bliss' approach,
Provides him happiness.

The Check ups

Introduction

By the time my husband needed medication and dietary intervention, to help cope with the changes taking place in him, our communication was becoming more difficult. I use the word 'our' as opposed to 'his' as communication is always a two way thing.

My husband may have found it harder to express himself due to physical. cognitive, and emotional problems, but I also found it harder to listen due to my own tiredness and confusing the signals being given by him. Couple with that my need to adapt my ways of talking; listening; intuitively knowing things, and also change habits of a lifetime (talking fast/doing everything at 100 miles per hour – see 'The Rushed Hush').

If you have read my poem 'The Cocktail' you will have already gathered I hold a suspicion of drugs being dished out without a lot of thought to their side effects. Look at any warning leaflets and labels given with medicines or supplements and you will see any number of potentially harmful physical and psychological changes which may occur as a result of taking.

It's all very well if we can feel and express the side effects in ourselves but what if we couldn't because of our disease masking them? Or worse still... What if we could feel/sense changes but have no way of getting it across to someone as we can't communicate our physical feelings or worries? Without being able to say "STOP" the unintentional torture goes on!

When giving my husband new medicines and supplements I took pains to chart as much as possible his reactions/changes (temperature; bowel and bladder movements; skin changes; irritability; sleep patterns etc, etc). However, it would have been wise to have pre-empted things by asking for a full blood and allergy test before it got to the point where I was having to second guess if my husband might be reacting to/allergic to what was being introduced to his body.

Take a simple - normally harmless - thing like milk for instance... To help weight gain we were given a milk based protein drink. Overnight my husband was being filled with a high dose of milk and minerals etc. He had not expressed any intolerance before when drinking milk but that was not at the same quantity. A drop of milk in his hot beverages and a small amount with his cereal etc. I did wonder after a while when he showed a rash if he had an intolerance to cow's milk. Should I have switched to goats milk boosting the lack of calories in another way? Wouldn't it be great if those at risk of HD were given a full health and allergy screening as part of their general well-being checks at – say – eighteen?

And then there's the matter of blood tests. Because my husband had been so healthy before HD took hold, and not needing blood checks previously, we found there was no recorded base-line data on what his normal blood counts would be in areas such as sodium; potassium; creatinine; calcium; alkaline phosphotase; gamma glutamyl; white blood count; red blood count; albumin; globulin etc. Changes in such areas are vital to giving clues to what may be disturbing a body and what needs treating and/or balancing.

There are 'normal' ranges which are used to try measuring whether a person has a particularly higher or lower count than should be expected but it differs from person to person where they may naturally be higher or lower anyway much like body temperature. What about the changes to blood with regards to medicines and supplements? Unless all introduced toxins and dietary changes were screened out it would never be easy to see what is 'normal'

There are other things to consider... When the disease had progressed to the point where blood tests might be needed for this and that, my husband had developed a fear of needles and nurses in general. This made it hard to do tests and extremely distressing for him. I wish we had at least a file showing what my husband's system was like before HD started taking over, and before I started giving him Tetrabenazine; protein drinks; cod liver oil; creatine; pure cacao etc etc. That could have reduced the amount of tests and saved time for someone so vulnerable and terrified at what was happening to him.

It's a simple, little tablet,
And it's there to help your pain,
But that tablet in your tummy,
Has set off your sweats again.

And the food that I just gave you,
Whilst it won't do this to me,
Will because it's so abundant now,
Cause you a rash or three.

Our confusion doesn't help us,
When you try to tell me "Stop!"
But I miss the vital signals,
As blood pressure starts to drop.

And the doctor looks at me for clues,
His records do not state,
If your vital signs are up or down,
Or just your normal rate?

So in dark we keep on working,
And the needles scare you so,
But without the map to plot our start,
We don't know where to go!

The Denial

Introduction

The Denial tries to convey "standard psychological denial". Here the person knows something is wrong but, understandably, makes excuses for everything so as to put off the likely confirmation of what they fear. In this case HD.

Self-denial using excuses and laughing it off is outlined in this poem. I have previously spoken of my aiding my husband's denial. It is crushing to tell someone you think the symptoms have started. I saw the signs several years before my husband finally went to see his GP.

Whilst I was miles away at work one day my husband accidently set our kitchen on fire. It was only mercifully a small fire, and he did manage to put it out with no harm to himself and just a burnt out rubbish bin and hole in our industrial (yes industrial) flooring. The episode shook us both up when thinking what could have happened not just to him but our neighbours given we were in a block of flats. It was at that point we both had to accept it was time to face up to the reality of needing outside help.

Denial itself is not straightforward. In the next poem – The Unawareness - I cover 'organic denial'.

There is a thin line between denial and unawareness and I am not sure which side of the line I could have placed my husband on if truth be known. At the time though... all I could see was that he was intent on avoiding the issue.

She's bumping into the chair again,
"Who put that there?" she jokes.
Walks past the rug she burned last night,
When dropping several smokes.

"I needed a new one" she says to herself,
As she's putting it in the bin bag.
"At least I know now the smoke alarm works",
She laughs as she's lighting her fag.

The neighbours chat in garden next door.
She can see they are looking her way.
"Nosey sods" she says under her breath walking in,
As she picks up her tea on the tray.

CRASH!!! goes the china as tea tray is dropped.
The neighbours jump over the wall.
"We're calling an ambulance, like it or not!"
"It's everyday now that you fall."

The Unawareness

Introduction

This poem was titled 'The Denial (Hard)' in my original book. It was to outline 'organic' denial as opposed to 'standard psychological denial' where a person is intentionally in self denial. The previous poem was originally called 'The Denial (Soft)' to differentiate a little.

In the process of looking up data for checking my sources I came across an interesting article titled.

'Understanding Behaviour in Huntington's Disease by Dr. Jane Paulsen
    Denial, Unawareness'

In it Dr Paulsen writes:

'Denial in an individual with HD is common. There are at least two reasons that denial can occur in HD. Commonly, denial is considered a psychological inability to cope with distressing circumstances.

We often see this type of denial in cases such as loss of a loved one (denial that they are gone), terminal disease, serious illness, or injury (i.e. denial of cancer or HD diagnosis). This type of denial, however, typically decreases over time as the individual begins to "face reality".

In contrast, individuals with HD often suffer from a lack of insight or self-awareness.

They are unable to recognize their own disabilities and are unable to evaluate their own behaviour.

This type of denial is sometimes called organic denial and is a condition that may last a lifetime. Given that we typically assume that denial is under the control of the individual, the term may not be useful for persons with HD suffering from this organic type of denial. Therefore, we recommend that "unawareness" be used to describe this behaviour in HD.'

The assumptions made, that the person actually has control, hit home. In view of this I thought it only right that I change the title to reflect better what may be happening.

He'd lost count at the number of times,
He'd said where they were going.
She asked again, confusion plain,
Frustration and anger growing.

He counted to ten, and said again,
"We're going to see the GP."
She threw down her bag, and as she lost her rag,
"Now why would he want to see me?"

"FOR GOD'S SAKE WOMAN,
There's something wrong!"
"Why can't you see it,
The signs are so strong?"

She took off her coat,
And sat on the chair.
"NOTHING'S WRONG WITH ME!"
"I'M NOT GOING ANYWHERE!"

The Panic Button

Introduction

In this poem I've tried to outline the underlying fear that those with a positive result for HD must be feeling. No matter how brave they may try to appear for others' sakes, it must be so hard having a black cloud placed over your head.

Sitting wife down, he passes a glass,
It's only half past four.
She takes a sip, and looks at clock,
Seems ominous that's for sure.

He goes on to tell her, what doctor has said.
For her too, first news of HD'!
She's shocked as she hears, confronted with fears,
Thinking 'What will this all mean to me?'

He then reassures her, acting the man,
That they've years yet, before it takes hold.
He then goes to tell her, one by one,
How the symptom signs they might unfold.

He labours the point, how she's not to panic,
A point he seems eager to make;
But she's quick to see, that this talk's not for she,
He's making it for his OWN sake!

The Innocent Answer

Introduction

Time and time again I read of people not knowing until they have made life decisions that a hereditary condition is lurking in the background.

Here we see a mother having to come to terms with hearing devastating news which may not only impact on her life but on that of her child. Suddenly her whole life and that of her husband will be turned upside down.

"What will I be when I grow up?"
The young boy asks his dad.
"Big and strong and happy my boy"
The father tells his lad.

The mother pulls her magazine,
Much closer to her head;
She's hiding tears of sorrow now,
On hearing what was said.

She hasn't even told the dad,
The secret she can't hide;
She's just discovered Huntington's,
Was on her father's side.

The father puts his son to bed,
"Now what were you going to say?"
She puts down mag, face tear stained now;
"I'll tell you about my day."

The Teacher

Introduction

In this poem I've again approached the subject of the juvenile strain of the illness (JHD). Although rare, HD does affect children. Without the recognition of HD, even in their own families where it may not have been openly talked about, who knows how many Melindas there are out there?

He picks up the work book, takes his pen;
Melinda's got that wrong again.
"It's such a shame" pops into his head;
Once 'Top of Class' she's last instead.

The change in her, it's hard to place,
Not just her work, but in her face.
She used to be a happy child,
Now face is twitching, although mild.

He'll ask her parents to come in;
He thinks he's heard her father's sick?
He overheard girls teasing Mel,
By putting on a nervous tic.

He'll do some searching later on,
Could something be hereditary?
He's stunned at where his search has gone;
He's found the cause, it's JHD!

The Teenager's Awakening

Introduction

This poem touches on the secrecy within families. There are still many people out there unaware of the potential time bomb ticking away in their bodies. With the advent of the internet, and wider recognition of the condition, there are fewer places to hide. Good or bad thing? You decide.

A few months after writing this poem, an article appeared in the HDA Newsletter. It was written and submitted to the HDA by a young lady who wanted to share her experience of hearing about HD with others. Felicity was just eleven when she wrote the following article.

I have reproduced the article alongside this poem as I thought it was important to balance the stark reality and shock portrayed in my poem against being open with children from the outset. I am sure everyone will agree that Felicity is a remarkable young lady!

'Telling Kids by A Kid

My name is Felicity, and I am eleven years old. *In 2008, I found out that my Nan had Huntington's disease. I had just turned ten, when my Dad told me. I have recently found out more about HD and I am very interested to find out more as I have a 50% chance of getting it when I am older.*

I am so very glad that my Dad told me as I would hate to not know something about my Nan, as I am close to her. Our family has coped with it well, and so have I. There's only one thing; my cousins do not know about my Nan, because that was my Auntie's decision not to tell them. I respect her opinion greatly, but I prefer to know. Personally, I feel it is wrong to not know about something that has happened, as they also have 50% chance, the same as me.

My Dad has explained everything to me about HD, so I am quite aware of what happens. He has made many friends over the HD Message Board, who I have also met. Everyone is very friendly, and I have also learnt many things from them.

Some people find it hard telling their children if a member of their family has HD, or may not want to tell them at all. Personally, my opinion (as a child), is to just tell them the truth; children are smarter that you think, and can sense things quite easily. I feel the best way is, like how my Dad told me, just tell them little bits at a time, let it sink in, soon they will start to think about what you have said, they will ask questions and all you need to do is tell them the truth. Do not add any other information, as they will ask you what they want to know. Don't be frightened of telling your kids, they have a right to know.'

The father of the young lady is DH. The same person who inspired me to write this book in the first instance. He is rightly very proud of Felicity, especially as she wrote and submitted her article to the HDA without any input from him whatsoever. He only found out about it after the event.

His future looked bright,
But that was before,
He heard conversations,
Behind the closed door.

His parents were crying,
He didn't know why,
He heard some parts clear though,
Like "HD" and "die".

And later that night,
With laptop in bed,
He Googled in private,
Words 'HD' and 'dead'.

Reality dawned,
Now all became clear;
His Grandma's strange movements,
'Hereditary.....FEAR!

The Driver

Introduction

Under UK law the Driver and Vehicle Licensing Agency (DVLA) requires that holders of licenses with the HD gene inform them upon becoming symptomatic. Forcibly stripping away a persons' independence is such a hard thing to do even if it is inevitably for their own safety as much as others.

This poem touches on the added dilemma facing families whose livelihood depends on driving. Even disclosure of 'at risk' status may cause all manner of problems.

As with a number of areas affecting those with HD and their families, the HDA produce a very useful Fact Sheet entitled 'Huntington's Disease and Driving'. Available direct from the HDA, or online at www.hda.org.uk.

He did 'The Knowledge' years ago,
His black cab is his pride.
Had many a star in back of cab,
All glad to take his ride.

The freedom of the road his love,
His streetwise savvy too.
He's earned a good rate working hard,
The bad fares have been few.

Then suddenly he heard his bruv,
"Isn't doing well."
His Mrs and his bruv's wife cry,
Though neither bird will tell.

Just why the sudden misery?
His Mrs, she won't say.
And how come she's been looking up,
The bleedin DVLA?

The Bucket List

Introduction

In the 2007 film 'The Bucket List' two terminally ill men go on a road trip to do the things they want to do before they 'kick the bucket'. Whilst learning you have the HD gene is never an easy thing to cope with... sometimes being faced with what may be an early end gives you the opportunity to appreciate the here and now more.

From our own Bucket List we managed to visit places like Florence, Rome, Paris, Barcelona, St Tropez, among other European destinations under our own steam or on cruise liners. We spent my husband's fortieth birthday in Boston Massachusetts. We celebrated our tenth wedding anniversary year with a cruise package combining travelling on the Orient Express and flying on Concorde! We went to the Grand National at Aintree and even climbed Mount Snowdon (by train I have to add). We didn't get to Egypt, Mexico or New Zealand but still... It was pretty good going don't you think?

The majority of the above was done before my husband became seriously symptomatic but I know that without the threat of HD possibly being on the radar we might just as easily have settled for putting things off until tomorrow. For some people tomorrow never comes. As the saying goes... "You never regret what you did... only what you didn't do".

He's just heard he is HD Plus,
He's sitting in a bar.
His mate's rushed over for support,
He's had to come so far.

It's closing time, his mate's in tow,
To make sure he's alright.
Both back at flat, the cans come out,
They put the world to right.

The conversation turns to death,
But not an ounce of sorrow.
They're making lists of what to do,
They'll start first thing tomorrow.

Places to go, and things to do,
So grateful to his friend.
Joint 'Bucket List' to be fulfilled,
Together til the end.

Section 4

Family
Values

Whether we are related by blood,
Or just by association,
I share your hope, your dreams your fears,
Your anger and frustration.

Introduction to Section 4

Family Values

By its nature, HD will have a far reaching impact on family members, loved ones and even friends. In this Section I have tried to bring out some of the interrelationship angles.

A number of the poems in other Sections could have quite easily slotted in here. Indeed, as with other Sections, poems from here could have slotted in elsewhere. Take 'The Best is Yet to Be' for example. I did originally have that under 'Adapt and Survive'. I thought it fitted well with the notion that we were being asked to consider ourselves as Old Age People (O.A.Ps) in some respects and maybe we would have been better off adapting in that way? I moved the poem as it had a whole new resonance when my husband died.

The 'Ripple Effect', 'Quality of Life' and 'The Normality' were written especially for the HDA as an exercise where they were presenting on the quality of life for families with HD at a World Conference. I wanted to reinforce it is important to recognise just how far reaching a holistic approach to treating, and supporting the family as a unit, could be!

The Lost Generation

Introduction

The following poem sets the scene of a young person growing up in a home where a parent is HD symptomatic. In it I have tried to convey what might be the loneliness experienced by the teenager, and how the dynamics of the family unit will have been changed by HD. The girl not only seems to have lost her father but her mother and her own childhood too.

Lucy is crying out for emotional and practical support but is unlikely to get that within the home. Not her mother's or her father's fault but who can she turn to who would understand?

There are a number of Young Carer projects, and they do a wonderful job. However, Lucy would probably learn sooner or later that at eighteen she can take steps towards finding out if she too has the HD gene, and all that testing brings with it whether she tests positive or not. Another dimension of stress placed upon young shoulders.

It was recognised there is little by way of coordinated tailored support and reference points for young people in the HD community. With this in mind, the HD Youth Organisation (HDYO) has been formed. HDYO will be the first organisation to specifically support young people from the HD community not just in the UK but internationally.

It will provide support, information, and educational videos about HD along with young people's experiences and support forums available in a variety of languages. The launch of the HDYO website is expected to go live by late 2011. Find the HDYO at **www.hdyo.org**

Putting on her blazer as she leaves home for her classes,
Lucy kisses daddy's head whilst stroking as she passes.
Daddy doesn't smile at all, or conversation start,
Lucy closing door behind her, sadness in her heart.

School is over, Lucy home, she goes straight up the stairs,
Mum is chatting to the doctor, daddy unawares.
Lucy knows she's not included, mum thinks she's too young,
Yet shortly after doctor leaves her day is just begun.

Helping with the tidying she makes them cups of tea,
And listens to her mothers' day whilst trying to watch TV.
She's told her mum her day was fine, she didn't want to add,
To her mother's stressful day by saying it was "bad".

Feeding daddy, wiping spills, to give her mum a break,
Lucy counts the tablets out, which hopefully he'll take.
Lucy broaches asking mum "what did the doctor say?"
"Nothing you need worry about" then mum just walks away.

Tired she goes up to her room, her homework to be done,
Double Science class today, genetics wasn't fun!
HD covered, cold as science, little do they know,
Just 14 she's tired of HD, nowhere she can go.

The Sibling

Introduction

This poem tries to convey how people at risk of developing the disease have different approaches to coping with not knowing. Some need to know their fate whilst others cannot face up to testing for the gene even though there is just as much chance they might be negative.

Here I also touch again on diagnosis by proxy. In essence, if one sibling tests positive he/she almost certainly confirms their parent is also HD positive and the others are confirmed as being at risk whether they wanted to know or not!

Both have grown up, to live with HD,
Their grandpa and aunty affected.
They know that their dad is at risk as well,
But attempts to discuss are rejected.

One sibling is eager to know of her fate,
The other is keen to ignore.
One feels that a family and children can wait,
But the other is hungry for more.

The answer is simple to those looking in;
Why doesn't the sibling just test?
But even the route to have testing begin,
Will open a whole hornet's nest.

The laid back sibling is quick to remind her,
It's not only your life at stake;
If you have the gene, then you know that will mean,
It's dad's and my heart too you'll break!

The Survivor's Guilt

Introduction

Survivor's guilt is now a recognised condition. It occurs where a person perceives they have done wrong and should feel guilty at surviving a traumatic event when others did not make it. The event can be mortal or even non-mortal situations. As inheriting HD is as simple as the toss of a coin, it is inevitable that those who do not inherit it will question why they were one of the 'lucky' ones.

This poem uses the non-identical (Dizygotic) twin scenario. There are a number of non-identical twins where HD has only affected one twin. Interestingly, for cases of HD in identical (Monozygotic) twins, there is evidence to show the timing of onset of disease may be affected by environmental factors such as smoking, thus suggesting there are steps people can take in lifestyle to help delay onset.

Source: Monozygotic twins discordant for Huntington disease after 7 years. **Friedman JH, Trieschmann ME, Myers RH, Fernandez HH.**

The test results in with a 'negative' stated,
To all looking on, she should feel elated.
Big smile on her face as she walks out the door,
And gives a thumbs up sign, she'll be back no more.

Now entering home, but what can she say?
They had no idea where she went to today.
She sits on the sofa and cuddles her mum,
Seems wrong to feel happy, she's luckier than some.

She moves from the sofa, she goes to make tea,
She passes her twin who shows signs of HD.
And later that night when she's all on her own,
She cries in her pillow, her grief can't be shown.

They once shared a womb, so how can this be,
At the toss of the coin, it chose him and not me?
A short spell of happiness, now filled with sorrow,
Though guilt overcomes her, she'll tell them tomorrow,

And very next morning, she takes mum aside,
Relief overwhelming, the tears of joy dried.
As all too soon after, the twin staggers in,
Both women look up, and excuses begin.

They know he'll feel happy, his sister is free,
But deep down inside he'll think "why was it me?"
So nothing is said, as the times' never right,
They'll keep their guilt hidden, til he's out of sight.

The Grandparent

Introduction

In this poem I have tried to touch on loss of family.

In many families, whether they be affected by HD or not, there are cases of family members being kept apart for a variety of reasons. Here we can see a differing of opinion on what would be best for the children and the grandparent.

The "cruel to be kind" line conveys not only trying to protect the grandchildren from seeing their grandparent so ill, but protecting them from seeing how they themselves may end up.

Visiting time in the nursing home,
The families of others arrive.
She had her hair brushed, luncheon was rushed,
And the wheelchair is pushed to the Drive.

The car pulls up, and her son climbs out,
She's hoping her grandkids will follow.
His wife steps out too, but no kids follow through,
She gives a false smile, masking sorrow.

They spend the next hour in the garden;
The others' grandchildren at play.
She's not seen her own for many a year,
She wishes it wasn't this way.

The kids are at home with their aunty,
Their dad's pleas all being in vain;
The women decided, 'be cruel to be kind',
And they'll never see Grandma again.

The Infrequent Daughter

Introduction

Here I have broached the hard subject of us carers really knowing what our charges want. There's a fine line between what the person themselves want, and what the carer thinks is best for them. That is true of any carer situation but, with HD and the tendency at times for irrational thinking, there is even more danger in dismissing the person's real wishes and needs. After all... as a tired and frustrated carer who was to say I was the one thinking clear and my husband was not? Sometimes I did wonder...

Visiting time, the Home's not bad,
It keeps him safe and looking well.
The Garden and the rooms are large,
The one before was small as hell.

His daughter smiles, she's pleased as punch,
She feels she's made a brilliant choice,
But what she doesn't see is this,
Her father misses that one voice.

For all the room and flowers there,
His favourite carers' far away,
And though his daughters' tried to care,
This isn't where he wants to stay.

She listens to him asking her,
To let him go back, can't stay here.
Dismissing him as HD talking,
She'll come back later, in the year.

The Quality of Life

Introduction

This poem tries to emphasise the need to look at the affect of illness on the whole family group. It's fair to say any illness one person has will have a knock on effect for those close. However, with its hereditary issues and the complexity of the illness (physical, psychological and emotional), by treating peoples' needs in isolation the health service are likely to be wasting resources.

Back from the Doctors,
With Pills for HD.
Not just the patient,
But whole family!

There's dad with the gene,
And son who's depressed.
There's mum who can't sleep,
And daughter who's stressed.

The powers on high,
Do not seem to think,
Of savings they'd make,
If they just made the link!

The link ... The core focus,
Their Quality of Life;
The effective way forward,
For man, child and wife!

The Ripple Effect

Introduction

This poem was written as one of three for the Huntington's Disease Association (HDA) who were presenting at an international conference on HD. The focus of the talk was the quality of life for families with HD and I wanted it to pay tribute to their work. Without such organisations totally funded by charity, and to whom I hope to help raise funds for by publishing this book, many would go under!

When the HD pebble is thrown,
It doesn't gently fall.
Your whole gene pool feels ripples,
The hardships shared by all.

With its linear path of destruction,
The chance of escaping is poor;
Even if not directly it's passed on to you,
It's still likely you're victim for sure.

But that doesn't mean it's reflected,
That the family's needs are all met;
There is some hope for all those affected,
Though there's still a way to go yet.

And with this in mind thanks must be given,
To those who are paving the way,
To improve quality, for the whole family;
The societies like HDA.

Huntington's Disease Association Head Office
Neurosupport Centre, Norton Street, Liverpool, L3 8LR
Tel: 0151 298 3298
Fax: 0151 298 9440
email: info@hda.org.uk

The Normality

Introduction

Because of the constant drains on sufferers and carers the need for respite care is very important. However, there are very few places for families with HD to go to where the special equipment and knowledge of the illness is available.

When my husband's condition deteriorated to the point he was unable to weight bear, and needed care above and beyond what I could cope with on my own, I still wanted to give him some quality of life by having trips to look forward to.

To take carers on holiday with us, and finding suitable accommodation with hospital type beds and hoists etc, was near on impossible; yet separating me from my husband and sending him to a residential home for a week to give us both 'respite' was not an option. Any benefits would be short lived and I doubt either of us would have relaxed whilst the other was not there.

We needed to have a break together! We had always holidayed together in the past so why split us up now if it could be helped? The HDA came to the rescue again. They were able to recommend a place in Norfolk called Park House (a hotel run by the Leonard Cheshire Disability Trust). **www.parkhousehotel.org.uk**

Park House is not a hotel with just token wheelchair access and a few grab rails. They can provide the full range of equipment such that you would expect in a nursing home, with a nurse and carers on call to provide as much or as little assistance as required, whilst still maintaining the experience of a relaxing hotel. They even have a lovely silver service restaurant and bar and outside swimming pool. Activities and entertainment are laid on and they organise trips to the seaside, shopping etc.

We were lucky enough to be able to self-fund our first few trips and thereafter get partial support through my husband's NHS Continuing Care package. From speaking to other carers also staying at the hotel, it was incredible just how the amount of support given varied from one social service provider to another. Some people received no support, financial or otherwise towards their stay, and others received full support including transport.

It could be argued the above should have been inserted in my 'Quality of Life' Introduction. By having that type of respite available to us as a couple, I am sure we saved the NHS thousands of pounds in nursing home and carer fees. Those breaks gave us the strength to continue coping at home for a lot longer than we would have done I am certain.

The children playing on the beach,
The mother taking sun,
The father too on holiday,
A family having fun.

A common scene you'd like to think,
But look again, you'll see;
The father in a wheelchair,
One child with JHD.

They're at a special Centre;
But the wife has had to fight;
Resources are so scarce it's sad,
They are not there by right.

For one week only of this year,
They block out their HD,
And feel the thing they long to have,
That thing......? Normality!

The Touching Moments

Introduction

This poem was penned on a day when I managed to stupidly knock my head on the metal part of the ceiling track hoist when attending to my husband. I was emotionally overwhelmed by my husband's sweetness and concern for me.

At the time of writing my husband had cognitive difficulties; he was in a wheelchair; he was incontinent; he had weakening muscles in his mouth and tongue making speech harder and more frustrating for him by the day. Shall I go on...?

Although he had an unbearable illness he suffered it with no self pity or real bitterness towards anyone. That said...He would get angry and frustrated with himself and me at times, who could blame him? I am sure I would have been an unbearable patient in his shoes.

However, at 'late stage' he seemed to have resigned himself to his fate. It must have been so humiliating for him having to be looked after like a baby! As strange as it may sound there were times I'd have given anything for him to go back to the man he was when shouting and agitated as it meant he had fighting spirit even if it was me he was sometimes fighting.

Bending down to put on the pad,
I straightened myself up when done.
Head was raised and on metal I grazed,
A shout out of pain where it stun.

The fear on his face as he looked up at me,
But I smiled and just pushed hoist away.
"I'm fine" I said, whilst rubbing my head,
As I heard him slur "Are you Okay"

It was only a bump but it made us both jump,
And it frightened him much more than me.
As the evening progressed, the same question addressed,
There was hardly a mark I could see.

As I tucked him in bed, his eyes fixed on my head,
Again he slurred was I "okay?"
It was touching to see, that he still cares for me,
When his own life is ebbing away.

'The Best Is Yet To Be'

Introduction

At the time of writing this poem (November 2009) I had some paperwork to look at. It was an application for consideration for "Extra Care Sheltered Housing".

Basically it was the equivalent of a retirement home with a warden and carers. In principle it sounded great but the normal criteria was that you had to be aged over 60, and that would have been the average age of the residents. Because of our circumstances, people thought we might be better placed there. We were both 48 at the time. They say "Life begins at 40". Then again... those last few years gave us precious time alone at home together which a lot of couples never get to achieve.

'Grow old along with me!
The best is yet to be';
It's clear when Browning, wrote those lines,
He hadn't met HD!

Meant to retire together,
Married same age as me;
We both envisaged a company clock,
And a bungalow by the sea!

In our forties and home together,
O.A.P.s we've become before time.
We cannot do 'fun', or hols in the sun,
Our mates they are all in their prime.

But there's one thing we will have forever,
And our friends will one day come to see,
That we may not have grown old together,
But our time was the best it could be.

Section 5

Adapt
and
Survive

When the Russian Roulette of the HD bullet,
Is aiming to shoot to kill,
Sometimes it's best to keep ducking and diving,
Rather than keep standing still!

Introduction to Section 5

Adapt and Survive

Every case of HD differs from one person to another. For some it seems to manifest itself more physically, and for some it's the change in mental capacity that seems to be the dominant trait.

The majority of the poems in this Section touch on the psychological changes. It's not always easy getting support to cope with the physical changes but I tended to find because it was easier to measure/demonstrate the affect in physical terms, such as difficulty in walking, holding a knife and fork etc, there was easier access to help in managing these changes from people like Occupational Therapists.

When it came to psychological changes, for my own part at least, I found there was little if any professional support. Take Obsessive Compulsion Disorder (OCD) for instance. No one was going to walk in with an adaptation to help me structure my husband's thought processes. Sure, they could understand it occurs and sympathise but not bring anything to the table to help us.

With that in mind, I found researching and finding reassurance that it was a symptom of HD helped in some ways. I was then able to reign in my emotional reflexes to a degree and tell myself "He can't help it... it's the disease and not him!" "It's not me imagining this and it's not my fault, it's just the way things are!"

I would be lying if I said that always worked but it helped to the point where I could adapt my own psychology. I virtually became a 'Stepford Wife' doing things just to save on the hassle of arguing. I would also pre-empt things... such as making sure a task was done at the exact time or in an exact way my husband liked to stop confusion and confrontation.

Ultimately, I adapted to fit in with the strange Planet HD, rather than expecting HD to fit in with Planet Earth. Unfortunately, the rest of Planet Earth was still very much grounded but in our own little home, especially towards the end, it was me and my husband against the World; not against each other. Had I not adapted I don't think I could have survived!

The OCD Plea

Introduction

Obsessive Compulsive Disorder (OCD) is now a relatively well known illness. It can form a big part of HD and can be infuriating when there is no rational explanation for why certain things have to be done at all, or done a certain way, and the world seems to revolve around trivial things.

That said...However hard it may seem, challenging the behaviour makes life even more frustrating for the observer and distressing for the sufferer who cannot help it when all is said and done. I admit it took a while for me to get there but, from my own personal experience, sometimes it is best not to question... just accept and go along with it.

It's also worth noting where some HD patients like and need routine, OCD can actually helps the carer as it structures the day and helps planning. Of course... chances are the fixation will be about something else after a while but as long as you try to recognise a pattern you may be able to look for triggers and work around them.

I would recommend reading John Harding's 'One Big Damn Puzzler'. The central character, William, suffers from OCD and comes into contact with many other sufferers.

'William's problem was Obsessive Compulsion Disorder... The way it worked for William was that he was plagued by unwanted thoughts that filled him with overwhelming anxiety that could only be alleviated by certain comforting rituals the practice of which would somehow – magically and illogically – ward off the things he feared.'

Obsessive Compulsive Disorder,
Just another symptom we get.
The rituals we need, within our lives,
Particular needs to be met.

My partner just don't understand it,
She thinks that I'm being a pain.
Doesn't she care, that by placing that there,
I must start this all over again?

The socks go on after the trousers,
The shirt goes on after the shoes.
It's not like she'll die, if she doesn't know why,
This particular order I use.

So why does she still go on moaning?
It's not her who has this HD.
The rituals are my way of coping,
So why can't she just let me be?

The Stuck Record

Introduction

Perseveration is described as 'the tendency of an idea, impression, experience, etc. to persist or recur, or of an individual to continue a particular mental activity without the ability to shift easily to another at a change in stimulus'. In Psychiatry terms it is, 'the persistent and pathological repetition of a verbal or motor response, often seen in organic brain disease....'

Source: www.yourdictionary.com

Here is just one example of perseveration. I have deliberately cut this to three parts as "What's that thing?' gets annoying to read after a while. In real life though that question could have gone on for hours!

"What's that thing?" she asks her daughter,
"What's what thing?" daughter replies.
"What's that thing?" she asks her daughter,
Daughter's now rolling her eyes.

"What's that thing?" she asks her daughter,
Daughter's trying to hold back,
"What's that thing?" she asks her daughter,
Daughter's primed now for attack.

"What's that thing?" she asks her daughter,
Daughter's calm now, counted ten.
"That thing there" she points at water,
Brain's stuck record spins again.

The Impatient Patient

Introduction

There's a book called 'Hurry up and wait' written by Jimmy Pollard. It's a bible for all those caring for HD patients!

The 'Hurry up' element of Jimmy's book sums up one of the key characteristics of HD patients in that they psychologically do not understand how to wait anymore. The person can't help it.

I suppose it's the other side of the coin with OCD where we may not see why trivial things or rituals not carried out can seem unacceptable for the HD sufferer. Take for example my husband needing his drink of vodka and orange at exactly nine pm. Not before, not after, but at nine pm each night.

I might have been in the middle of doing something and have to stop and be ready for when the clock struck nine. In my husband's mind, what could be more important? Surely whatever I was doing could wait? It's not like I didn't know nine pm would be on its way is it after all? He had a point but that didn't make it less grinding...

In Section 8 'Time to Change' I have inserted an internet article I wrote back in November 2009 about my husband's fixation with clocks. Sadly his own time ran out too soon.

She looks at clock and counts the minutes,
Until it's half past three.
She knows 3:30 is the time,
She has her cake and tea.

The Carer's busy clearing up,
The mess made on the floor;
Been rushing back and forth all day,
She cannot take much more.

3:31 and comes the shout,
The anger lies beneath.
The Carer tries to block it out,
And swears through gritted teeth.

3:32 and sure enough,
She hears another shout.
The Carer holds her temper back,
THAT CLOSE from walking out.

The Reader

Introduction

My poem 'The Impatient Patient' is about how infuriating HD patients can be. This one was written to try and get across the other side of how rewarding it can be looking after a loved one and how hard it is for the person affected.

Whilst the majority of the poems have been written having looked at many peoples' tales of HD, this one was simply about me and my husband. He was still able to read a little bit as of Nov 2009. However, as every day passed by, his reading skills were diminishing but he tried his hardest to hide it.

Sometimes when my husband was struggling so hard to read an item such as sport, where he really wanted to know what was happening, I would make some excuse to read the article aloud. I could see he was relieved but embarrassed. I did my best to help him retain his dignity as each layer of independence was taken from him but it was only a matter of time...

I would like to add that even just a few months before my husband died we were still getting his eyes checked. When it was hard to get to the optician we used a home visit service (The Outside Clinic).
www.outsideclinic.com

The illness did not affect his eyesight. Whilst reading skills may have been diminishing, because of needing to concentrate more on word formation/ meaning, tiredness and poor posture as much as anything else, it should never be taken for granted eyesight and hearing themselves do not merit regular checks for a person with HD just as much as a person without.

He read the paper avidly,
But as the illness grew,
His reading skills were fading fast,
Nothing they could do.

But rather than admit defeat,
And take pleasure away,
She carried on regardless,
And bought the thing each day.

OK she had to turn the page,
His hands no longer able,
And then she had to fold it right,
To fit his bedside table.

From time to time she'd read aloud,
If struggling so she felt.
The little looks of gratitude;
Her heart would simply melt.

The Rushed Hush

Introduction

This poem was penned after reading a magazine article. It was about a woman who had died having suffered from HD. The article described her decline saying that she actually went blind, deaf and dumb because of the illness.

I was horrified to think her family may have simply assumed she had lost such faculties because they did not engage her in enough mental, sensual, aural and visual stimulation. In effect she would have been shut behind a wall of innocent negligence.

In my Introduction to 'The Reader' I highlight how my husband's faculties such as sight did not diminish with HD. His eyes slightly deteriorated through age, just as mine have done, but HD did not take away his ability to see, it simply made things harder for him in other ways. He could never in a million years have been described as blind, deaf or dumb!

I know first-hand how frustrating and time consuming it can be to look after someone with HD and how little knowledge there is out there about it both for families and the medical profession. To that end I can, to a degree, understand how easy it is to make such assumptions. That doesn't make it any easier to accept it happens.

Having said the above, I admit there were times in my frustration and despair it would have been easier to go into denial mode that my husband was still in there. I always tried to remind myself, no matter how hard it was to look after him, his time was running out and more precious than mine and I needed to make more of an effort for his sake. That included remembering to speak slower; take time to listen no matter how painfully slow things were and wait for a response.

Jimmy Pollard's book 'Hurry up and Wait' makes useful reading in terms of understanding HD behaviour. There are a number of exercises which help the carer better understand and empathise with how the patient's thinking is affected and why their comprehension may be compromised.

Please speak to me, I am not deaf;
Please show me flowers, I am not blind;
Please take the time to listen more,
I simply have a slower mind.

90

Please stay with me a moment longer,
Your time's precious, mines' more so;
Please try to talk a little slower,
I get confused lest you talk slow.

Please give me time to think a while,
It doesn't help when you cut in;
Please treasure silence, not fill void,
Please watch my lips till speech begins.

Please feed me love, it makes me stronger,
To fight this illness in my head;
Please care for me a little longer,
Your time is plenty, when I'm dead.

The Magic of Music

Introduction

Professor Edmond Chiu, as Senior Lecturer – University of Melbourne, gave a presentation on HD and noted "Our experience is that the Huntington's patient retains the ability to appreciate music right to the end. It may be that the part of the brain controlling music ability and music appreciation is not affected by Huntington's Disease. We don't know where that part of the brain is, but where ever it is they appreciate music. That is a very important part of their quality of life.'

This poem tries to reflect my own husband's continued love of music which seemed to stimulate his brain and generated much dialogue between us. A certain track or video would trigger memories and/or emotions. I found it important to have music around us and listen out for familiar tracks where my husband would want to talk about the group, a concert we went to etc (Rock or eighties music in our case) and even if he only got out a few words my giving him my attention, and adding a little bit at strategic moments to show I was listening/appreciated his thoughts seemed to bring him back to normality.

He's 10 years into symptoms,
The illness taking hold.
A couple of infections,
Has helped to make him old.

The frame once large and muscular,
Has since been taking flack.
A special chair's been purchased,
To help support his back.

And whilst to most observers,
He's not the man he was,
His friends all know it's not the case,
He's still the same because.

Because when they play music,
When hard rock fills the air,
The change in him amazing!
Their old mate's sitting there.

The Tooth Fairy

Introduction

Having previously written about the need to ensure regular health checks, I am all too familiar with the difficulties in getting someone with HD to general appointments let alone the dentist.

Visiting the dentist strikes fear in many people and a natural reluctance and phobia in the first place doesn't help. With HD there are the added complications of not only getting to the dentist, but in being able to examine properly when there. Getting into the chair itself; keeping still; keeping the mouth open; swallowing/aspiration into the lungs of foreign matter making the use of dental equipment at best awkward, and at worst dangerous, etc, etc.

Much of the above applies to other checks it is true but in terms of oral hygiene and dental care there is much more to it than quality of life.

Rikki's Story', reproduced in Section 8, tells the tale of a family trying to cope with Juvenile HD. Here are some extracts:

'... Rikki couldn't open her mouth to eat or drink. Overnight, her jaw clenched tightly shut. It took me 2 hours to get a couple of ounces of water into her via a gap in her teeth with a baby's medicine syringe...'

'Hindsight is a wonderful thing isn't it? I look back now and feel very sure that the sudden over night jaw clenching was to do with dental problems. But at the time, I only saw what was in front of me...that Rikki could no longer eat or drink. After Rik had been PEG fed we noticed a swelling on the side of her face...a sure sign she had an abscess. Rik was put on antibiotics and the swelling went down.'

I was lucky enough to be able to get domiciliary dental checks for my husband where it was too impractical for me to take him to the dentist all the time. Through getting to know and trust the Team in the comfort of our own home, we were able to get my husband to trust them enough to be wheeled to the Surgery when needing a filling even at late stage. He remained in his wheelchair throughout the procedure, the Team were amazing with him, and was the perfect patient.

Domiciliary dental services are, I suspect, few and far between but it is always worth making enquiries explaining in depth how hard it is for the patient and carer, and also how lack or oral care can have such a devastating impact on sufferers.

Brush twice a day, the dentists say,
Two minutes up and down.
Will help you style, a beaming smile,
Instead of grumpy frown.

But what when more than vanity,
Is driving mouth's attention?
The simple task of brushing teeth,
In need of intervention

The hands that cannot hold a brush;
The mouth that will not play;
The dental wash that's swallowed,
Where it's meant to wash away.

It's hard enough to feed you now,
But still I try in vain,
Not seeing that the root of cause,
May stem from oral pain.

You can't convey what I can't see,
Your pain from hot and cold;
The dental visits had to cease,
When HD took its hold.

The Hunger

Introduction

In this poem I have tried to bring out how lonely the sufferers must be when their families and friends block them out from social interaction. It's true that communication is difficult but it must be so lonely shut within your shell, watching others live life as though nothing had changed.

The Sunday lunch setting reminded me how torturous it must be to have your senses stimulated by food and yet, because of swallowing difficulties (or maybe even dental issues given the previous poem), all you will be fed is unappetising pureed food or a tasteless milk protein drink!

Incidentally... When looking into the pros and cons of tube feeding (Percutaneous Endoscopic Gastroscopy – PEG) in order to evaluate better the quality of life for my husband, I learnt that whilst PEG feeding would help deliver calories and nutrients, patients who could still swallow should be encouraged to eat small amounts for food normally for as long as possible.

Sitting in the lounge alone,
The radio playing low.
The family pop in now and then,
To say a quick hello.

In kitchen they are chatting,
The usual family bunch.
Tradition held for years and years,
Down mum and dads' for lunch.

The dad has taken on mum's role,
Not easy task he boasts.
A dab hand now with gravy,
And even matched her roasts!

They wheel her into dining room,
The part she's come to dread.
No plate piled high to share the food,
Milk protein drink instead.

The Corrupted Computer

Introduction

One of the Message Board members (Twamoons) posted up once about some very interesting guidance she was given in relation to her husband and how the HD brain might work. In essence, the specialist explained the brain was divided into shelves, and all the information we have gathered over the years is filed away on shelves. She said the HD person just took a little while longer to find which shelf, or part of the shelf, the information they were trying to find was on.

It makes sense... If we were to imagine our brain as a repository, and there are hundreds and thousands of shelves with everything we have ever learnt filed and archived neatly away, we would need some way of retrieving data in milliseconds for recall. Go on to imagine having all our thoughts catalogued and indexed on a super, dooper mega computer which has super fast automatic grabbers ready to find and retrieve any file we need in an instant. On top of that, you have new experiences and information needing to be catalogued and filed every day.

Then imagine that super dooper computer starts to get corrupted and the programme is getting slower and slower. Chances are, with new files being needed every millisecond (be it a question asked by someone or how do I do something?) the back-log of file requests would probably lead to a log jam. If the person were an organisation, reverting back to good old fashioned manual archiving and retrieving might be used until the computer could be trusted again.

It's no wonder people with progressive HD sometimes give up on trying to do the most basic of tasks and communication if having to access so many shelves, with no way of doing it fast enough, means they are put under immense stress!

"Mr Smith, would you like some milk in your tea?"
It's a simple question she's asking of me,
But I'm not sure if I should say "no" or say "yes"
And my cognitive programme's unable to guess

So I send off Bert, he's my man on the train,
To ride down my neurons to that part of brain,
It's the shelf labelled 'preference' but where can it be?
There's a million and one shelves that Bert can now see.

And the files on the shelves are stacked up so high,
That Bert heads back clueless, he'll not even try.
And the cups' handed over, fed up with the wait,
I sip the black tea which both Bert and I HATE.

The Brothers in Arms

Introduction

In this Section I thought it only right that I acknowledge the HDA and other HD Associations have also had to adapt in today's harsh economical climate.

In 2009 the four Huntington's disease charities throughout the UK and Southern Ireland came together to launch a unique Alliance through Huntington's Disease Awareness Week. The aim of the collaboration was to make as many people as possible aware of this disease and its devastating effect on whole families.

The new partnership is called 'The UK and Ireland Huntington's Alliance'.

Whether London, Belfast, Cardiff,
Whether Glasgow or Dublin;
The enemy we call HD,
Won't care which place you're in.

Across the regions far and wide,
Societies old and new,
Commit to standing side by side,
With so much more to do.

As the interest is ignited,
And Societies come to fore,
Linked together they're united,
Against the HD War.

As brothers in arms they're standing tall,
And fighting the War together;
The common purpose after all,
Is to stop HD forever!

Section 6

Low

Society

Look at me, what do you see,
And who are you to say,
That I should be, classed differently,
And treated in this way?

Introduction to Section 6

Low Society

Discrimination is natural. We all do it whether we like to admit to it or not. Many poems in this Section could have been written about any number of disabilities or vulnerable sections of society.

Discrimination can be born out of ignorance. Hopefully awareness initiatives will help to chip away discrimination. However, I can't help but feel when it comes to HD it gets more than its fair share of adverse discrimination and that its victims are penalised every which way...

Take insurance... Now the companies are aware HD has a genetic test which is a good indicator of someone's fate, they may have you over a barrel if there is a family history. In the case of a positive gene test, they can even legally discriminate in certain circumstances.

I have also included in this Section discrimination in the workplace not just for those with HD but in terms of getting back to work for carers like myself. The latter has become even more apparent during the bringing together of the old and new poems now that my husband has died.

'The Help' covers an area that will affect every one of us. Who will look after us when we get old and infirmed be it HD related or not? I have seen plenty of programmes that highlight negligence and abuse in care for the old and infirm which doesn't bode well.

I hasten to add neglect and abuse can take place in the patient's own home just as easily, if not more so, than in a nursing home where there are no regular checks or procedures in place to record and redress. I have touched on that in Section 7, 'The Tug of Love'.

The Insurance Salesman

Introduction

In October 2000 Britain became the first nation to approve the commercial use of gene technology to allow insurers to refuse cover, or to push up premiums for those born with genes that could lead to fatal conditions. HD was singled out as the only case allowed immediate discrimination because of the reliability of the test. This meant for a person having tested positive, insurers gained the right in certain circumstances to refuse to insure, or to legally load the premium to extortionate levels (300% has been cited).

So let's take a hypothetical scenario...

Let's say a person took the test at eighteen and tested positive. There are no signs of HD but he wanted to know if he had the gene. At twenty he applies for cover but has to declare a positive gene result and the cost of the insurance cover reflects this. At the same time his twenty year old neighbour has also applied for cover but he does not have any record of HD in the family. That's not to say he has no links to HD or any other potentially fatal disease, he just doesn't know about it yet. His policy costs 100% less.

The HD+ person pays the loaded cover pricing from day one but, where HD is not an exact science, he does not become symptomatic until in his sixties (known as 'Late Onset'). In those forty years before symptoms appear the person has led a HD free and health conscious life whereas his neighbour has not, and needs to draw on the cover much earlier.

It occurs to me there seems to have been no consideration of the fact that until symptoms start showing and presenting a problem ... the person with the HD gene may have the gene but does not have HD itself! It's no wonder this discrimination drives some people to delay testing where they feel it may compromise their right to be treated fairly and be refused mortgage cover etc.

Please note: As at time of writing this (March 2011) The Association of British Insurers (ABI) has a Code of Conduct stipulating rules which all its Members are obliged to follow. The Code sets out clear guidance where the use of genetic information may be used in calculating cover requirements. No Insurer can request an applicant take a genetic test for consideration of insurance. Set levels of values of policies dictate whether test results can be used in the assessment.

The HDA have prepared a Fact Sheet 'Advice on Life Assurance, Pensions, Mortgages etc.' which is available direct from the HDA on accessed through their website.

He's looking at the paperwork,
He's thinking of commission.
He'll reach his bonus target soon,
Just one more sale he's missing.

And this signed piece of paper,
Will take him to his score;
Be home in time for dinner,
So glad he chose this door.

But hold on, wait a minute,
What's she put on that bit?
'Genetic testing.. Huntington's',
He nearly has a fit.

He grabs the piece of paper;
Ignores her look so sad.
She thinks that we'll insure her life?
The woman must be mad!

The HD Shopping Trolley

Introduction

People with HD can take on as many as 5,000 - 7,000 calories a day without gaining weight. Maintaining a healthy weight is paramount but can be an uphill struggle especially when swallowing difficulties and risk of choking is high. Add to that we all know how hard it is to feel hungry when feeling ill and low.

Loading meals with calories by adding cream, butter and high fat produce may sound like a dream to some people but it is harder to keep on the weight than you might think! I mentioned in 'The Check Ups' I had my own worries that too much dairy produce was having an adverse affect on my husband but what were the alternatives?

Society is geared to weight loss and this is reflected in the food retail trade. It was getting harder by the day to think of ways to make mealtime more interesting and produce high calorie appetising food. Home-made soups with double cream were relatively quick and easy to make but even they started to get tedious for my husband towards the end.

There is, as always with HD, the other side of the coin though. Because of the energy used in simple day to days tasks for someone with HD there is often a stage where the sufferer is constantly hungry be it a physical need or a habitual desire where OCD may overtake the brains signals of being full.

It's never easy walking away from feeding someone who cannot feed themselves with a plate half or more full and wondering if they are still hungry but have stopped eating due to lethargy and fear of choking, or they are not hungry and to give more would be force feeding. Either way the carer may feel they are inadvertently being cruel.

I would often eat late night in private where I couldn't bear to think my husband was hungry but had no way communicating that to me, or that he would love to be eating what I was if only he could still eat normal meals. I also stopped eating food that gave off an appetising smell and look. My poem 'The Hunger' refers here.

A Saturday in Sainsbury's,
She's walking down the aisle.
The trolley fairly hard to push,
But still she has a smile.

The trolley piled up high with goods,
She looks at what she's bought.
It's drawing some attention now,
She understands their thought.

And as the checkout girl does scan,
She gives a funny look.
She wonders 'how comes she's so thin?
She ought to write a book!'

For in the shopping trolley,
It's non HDP's DREAM.
The chocolates, cakes and full fat meals,
The butter and the cream.

'Big Brother'

Introduction

Big Brother (UK) came to an end in 2010 but I dare say it will be back one day and the producers will be looking for other ideas. It wouldn't surprise me if they used a vulnerable section of society. It could be argued all the contestants have been mentally unstable already but with the HD Patients' (HDPs) cognitive and motor function problems alongside social awareness problems...

The Introduction above and poem below was written in 2009 when it was announced Big Brother was ending. I changed the wording slightly in 2010 to reflect the programme had ended. I am now updating this on 5th April 2011 and lo and behold, as I was doing an internet search to check my facts it was announced today Big Brother is to return in 2012!
Source – Guardian.co.uk 5th April 2011

That was incredibly spooky but I just hope and pray I am not psychic insofar as they run out of ideas during the 'five year contract' with Channel 5 and start filling the BB House with certain cross sections of an even more vulnerable society like some sort of disabled human HD fish tank.

I should really find something now to rhyme with Channel 5 but indulge me on this one please...

It's 2012 in London Town,
The crowds all scream and roar.
It's not the opening of the Games,
It's simply Channel 4.

BB is now back on the screen,
And how it's stooped so low.
The House is full of HDPs,
Their plights' a media show!

The pacing rooms relentlessly,
The outbursts of their rage;
The pulling hair and lack of care,
Like monkeys in a cage.

And yet the public still tunes in,
Will someone stop this thing?
A freak show for the masses,
But profit is the king!

The Wheelchair Outing

Introduction

The progression of HD often leads to the need of a wheelchair. My husband resisted using a wheelchair for many years even though his poor balance and tiredness meant he was prone to falls. I didn't exactly pressure him into using one, not just because it was another sign of loss of independence but it would have been harder for me too in many respects.

What I wasn't prepared for, when the time came, was the social stigma attached to wheelchair users insofar as becoming a kind of non-entity! In a weekly blog I wrote in 2008 I wrote about the first time I took my husband out in a wheelchair. It angered me how peoples' attitudes seemed to change overnight.

Like many examples in this book, this poem goes beyond HD as an illness and extends to disability and carers whatever their circumstances. The blog entry is extracted in 'One scoop of patronisation or two?' given in Section 8.

Walking down the High Street,
Hand in hand like lovers,
The couple blend into the crowd,
No different from the others.

As the years go by though,
His body having changed,
Has sadly meant a wheelchair,
Has had to be arranged.

Strolling down same High Street,
The woman now behind,
Her lover needing pushing,
Steep pavements so unkind.

Entering the bar now,
With awkward navigation,
People jump to open door,
Aware of situation.

"Thank you" says the man in chair,
When wheeled into the place;
"Welcome" say the helpers there,
But all avoid his face.

Carer get's the "Welcome" mouthed,
No looks at him they share,
Let's treat this fellow human being,
As if he wasn't there.

The Help

Introduction

It's fair to say, over the years, a better understanding and recognition of HD has resulted in better nursing home facilities for sufferers. Sadly there are still places where the care of those with HD, and I'm sad to say care of the vulnerable in general, leaves a lot to be desired.

My husband made me promise him I wouldn't put him in a home. I was fortunate enough to be able to keep him with me until the end. He died in his chair in our lounge with me holding his hand and it was a peaceful ending.

It was hard looking after him but we were luckier than many where we were allocated an adapted flat through Social Services and had a wonderful support system. The Community Rehabilitation Team in my Borough – Greenwich – came up trumps by being proactive as well as reactive. I should also mention that my husband's carers, initially provided through Social Services and then under NHS Continuing Care, were wonderful ladies who treated Steve with compassion and professionalism.

She sits in chair, her sloping frame,
The nurse runs by, no sound she hears.
She cannot speak the nurse's name,
The uniform, it disappears.

Her eyes look round for someone who,
May stop a while and notice how,
Her arm is twisted, cannot move,
Her eyes are filling, crying now.

Another patient sees her face,
And grabs the cleaner; holds her tight.
She shouts that "Irene needs a hand";
She gets shrugged off with "She's alright."

And so it goes for half an hour,
Til finally her family near.
And in a flash, staff rally round,
"Now Irene.... Let us help you dear".

The Prescription

Introduction

As time went by my husband needed more and more prescribed drugs, creams, protein drinks etc. We were not on income based benefits and, living in England*, we were told we had to pay for everything. The costs were escalating and although I bought pre-paid certificates it was another cruel expense for something that was no fault of ours.

I was aware some conditions merited instant waiving of charges and I considered it was unfair HD did not automatically come into the frame upon diagnosis, or at least when drugs and prescribed nutritional drinks were needed. I started making enquiries but was told at every turning HD was "Not on the list of exempt conditions".

After more investigations, and finally getting sight of the so called 'List of exemptions' when discussing the matter with the Department of Health, I found that my husband should not have been paying for his prescription for several years once he had deteriorated and become at risk of danger when leaving the house unaccompanied.

It was true that HD itself was not listed. However, what no GP or anyone else had done was to look beyond the names of illnesses and read the last qualification which states 'A continuing physical disability which means you cannot go out without help from another person.' If they had seen it, then all I can say is it was never asked of me if that would apply. The question was given on Form FP92A. In the circumstances, the NHS refunded the costs of my Pre-Paid Certificates but it was another battle I could have done without. HD is unjust enough as it is...

Perhaps we should move to Wales my love,
I think it could be wise,
We can't afford these spiralling costs,
And a different law there applies.

The man next door is able to work,
But he gets his meds for free;
It's sad he's diabetic my love,
But he's not like you and me.

We're stuck in this rut, and cannot work,
And we know life won't get any better,
But we're told again that your illness don't count,
According to this doctor's letter.

It CAN'T be right; I'm taking it further,
And finally we're getting somewhere,
A clause in the Form was missed my love,
As nobody spotted it there!

*UK Prescription charges as at 5th April 2011
England: £7.40 per item
Wales: No charge
Scotland: No charge
Northern Ireland: No charge

The Benefit Cheat

Introduction

I opted to put 'The Prescription' in this Section as I felt there was a social injustice issue in it. It occurred to me instead of assisting and wanting to enable those with HD and their families/carers to get financial support, there seemed to be a suspicion that everyone out there is just in it for what they could get. I shall resist the urge to comment on the pros and cons of the current changes in the benefits system as at April 2011.

In our case, the denial aspects of HD meant we did not claim for anything more than Job Seekers Allowance (JSA) or get any real support until actual diagnosis. This was despite it being acutely obvious the illness was taking hold.

At the time a specialist was seen, and blood was drawn (17th March 2005) my husband was on JSA and had been so since 2003. The poor man had been laid off many jobs, no doubt due to his performance getting worse, yet they did not know there was an underlying cause. He was still convinced someone would employ him until April 2005. I had to sit down with him at the Jobcentre and, with the help of his advisor who was by now aware of the HD explaining his struggles, tell my husband he would never work again. He was then put on Incapacity Benefit and I applied for Disability Living Allowance for him and later Carers Allowance for me when I had to cease work to look after him full time.

This poem is not about benefit cheats in the sense that society tend to think of... scroungers, spongers, fraudulent etc. Denial of HD can lead to support being withheld understandably as it has not even been claimed for. That's not to say it isn't much needed, it might be that it's a case of those in real need are being cheated of benefits, by reluctance to accept it is time...

The HD now affects his brain,
His office getting worried,
Relationships begin to strain,
His exit now gets hurried.

With wife aware his time is short,
And skills get more diminished,
She hasn't got the heart to say,
His working life is finished.

Their income now is cut in half,
They can't afford their pride,
He could apply for further help,
If HD weren't denied.

The benefits kick in at last,
When diagnosis made;
No mention though of all funds,
The system could have paid.

The Return to Work Interview

Introduction

This poem tries to convey the frustration held by many where society does not see "caring" of loved ones in the home as a job worthy of recognition. It's sad that when our loved ones die, and we no longer have a role, we not only have to cope with grief but have to start all over from scratch again.

It often means having given up careers and our own sense of identity. However, we have just had the toughest job in the world, somehow survived, but have nothing to show for it! The 'spotty youth' reference is there to highlight by definition those conducting the Job Centre interviews may be a lot younger than the person seeking work. They may not have the worldly wisdom on their side to recognize what sacrifice has been made by the person starting over, and what respect should be afforded to the person having been cared for.

I wrote this poem before my husband died. This edited section within the Introduction is being typed on 6th April 2011. I recently 'signed on' only to be told in a letter from the authorities that I will not receive any Job Seeker's Allowance. Their excuse was that I have not paid enough Class 1 National Insurance (NI) Contributions for tax years ending 2009 and 2010.

The NI contributions awarded when I was being given Carer's Allowance did not extend to Class 1, only Class 2. They do not count my giving up working to look after my husband full time and saving the country thousands in nursing home and care costs as worthy of recognition. It appears I joined the ranks of unemployed.

I was paid just over £50 per week Carer's Allowance for a 24/7/365 job for several years. All I have to show for it is a sense of immense pride and a five year gap in my CV which I am told makes me harder to employ. I 'signed off' on 4th April 2011, just a few weeks after signing on, when I was told I am not entitled to any support towards re-training to help me get onto the job market which has now moved on beyond my recognition.

Had I continued to attend the Job Centre according to my rejection letter, I may still have been entitled to my NI Stamp. I needed to show them sufficient evidence of focussing on getting a job with all the rejection that involves, alongside coping with grief and loss of my husband.

Until I do get a job I would rather live on the savings and pension lump sum released for my husband which will run out sooner rather than later at this rate. Probably a foolish thing to do but I am simply too disgusted to care about what the future may bring anymore!

She gave up work in 99,
To care for her poor dad.
Masters Degree was halfway through;
Promotion to be had.

She hasn't felt denied at all,
She's never felt regret.
The skills she's had to learn on job,
The challenges she's met.

She's been his nurse; his doctor; lawyer,
Admin person too.
Neuro researcher; OT; teacher;
Nothing she can't do!

The spotty youth in her Job Centre,
Looks at her C.V.
"So what you done these last ten years?
Hmmmmmmm, Nothing so I see."

The Boss Part (1)

Introduction

This poem is Part one of a two parter. It's clear that the workplace does not sit easy with those facing HD. The reference to HD being associated with 'High Definition' television highlights the ignorance and, as with the genetic testing scenario, once information is shared it cannot be taken back.

Time for Claire's Appraisal,
It was well overdue.
This time the boss became concerned,
At what he had to do.

The problem? Her performance,
Was clearly getting poor.
He couldn't understand it?
She'd been his 'rock' before!

So when it came to interview,
Her boss tried helping out.
"Are there any problems Claire,
That I should know about?"

"I have HD" Claire bravely said;
"Your telly?" came reply.
The ignorance slapped Claire in face,
And she began to cry.

The Boss (Part 2)

Introduction

This is Part two of a scenario where the workplace has learnt of an employee facing HD.

Employment rules have come a long way to guard against discrimination on the grounds of disability. However, it is still so hard when you feel you are not as valued as you were once.

Three months on from Appraisal,
And Claire has been moved on.
Her boss became so distant,
And things were feeling wrong.

He argued that her skill sets,
Were sadly now found lacking;
If not for Personnel's input,
He would have argued sacking.

So now Claire's sat in Post Room,
The only job they had.
Okay it is less daily stress,
But Claire is feeling sad.

She feels for all the years they shared,
He didn't want to know.
He couldn't handle her needs now,
Her boss just let her go.

Section 7

The
Dark side
Of
The Prune

If God exists, in any form,
The Devil must do too.
How else can I explain away,
What's happening to you?

Introduction to Section 7

The Dark Side of the Prune

I mentioned in the Introduction to this Book that my poems in this version went beyond what I would have felt able to submit to the HDA for inclusion in anything printed and distributed by them. The poems below illustrate where I was coming from as I tackle controversial areas such as euthanasia and death, and somewhat disgusting areas such as toileting. Hence the reference to Dark Side and Prune. I've also, rather clumsily, played with the Pink Floyd album title 'Dark Side of The Moon' where a big part of the Section relates to sleep disturbance. I came to dread the moon as it shone on the darker side of my husband's HD – 'Myoclonus'.

Many of the poems below have come direct from my own husband's progression of HD to some degree or another. All of the subject matters have been spoken about on the HDA Message Board, leaving me to feel I was not the only one wondering if certain aspects and feelings were normal, and that it was okay to talk about taboo subjects.

Hugh Marriott's book 'The Selfish Pig's Guide to Caring' was a turning point in my caring. It helped me realise many of my guilty feelings were normal and understandable. I was doing the best I could in extremely difficult circumstances, and I was not alone in being shell-shocked by the physical and emotional changes in my husband.

It also gave me more confidence to do my role and recognise I was a 'professional carer' just as much as anyone with an NVQ (actually, it has to be said, even more so) and I deserved to be respected for it. In essence, it was my job (albeit unpaid) and even the nastier sides of it should be accepted and handled to the best of my ability.

When I worked in an office I always tried to work by the rule that if I wouldn't be prepared to do something myself, I shouldn't expect anyone else to be prepared to do it. That helped me when it came to getting down to the nitty gritty (*or should that be shitty gritty*) parts of being a carer.

The first three poems in this Section talk about bodily functions. I expect it won't apply to every patient that they become so dependant, or maybe it will but no one talks about it enough for it to seem identified as an issue? Whatever the case, if we apply how we feel when our system is not working in harmony we surely can't ignore the impact it must be having on others who cannot express themselves fully.

Apologies in advance to anyone reading poems one to three whilst eating!
God knows what the poor proof reader of this is thinking...

The second two poems touch on patient abuse and the feelings of loneliness and lost love (myself being jealous of a toy cat for one thing). I had intended to do a number of other poems on relationship issues but, where I was needing to write them after my husband's death, I found the subject matter too stressful for a number of reasons. Maybe one day...

The next four cover what came to be the most tormenting for me to write at the time (all four before my husband died) but even more tormenting for me to read back now. My husband's most profound aspect of HD was when he would appear to be tortured in his dreams and kick and scream out in his sleep. He was always unaware of doing it.

The episodes were nightly for a few years and then tapered off before the end of his life. However, as they tapered off they were followed by other complications such as the first signs of pressure sores. At least when he was kicking about his circulation was good. At least when he was screaming out his facial muscles were exercised. I think my husband's restlessness in bed was extreme compared to others with HD but I can't be sure. Increasing his medication for a while (Tetrabenazine) did not help and I was reluctant to go down the route of him relying on sleeping pills.

In these poems I admit I felt it would be kinder for him to be dead than suffer as I felt he was doing. The thing is... My husband still had a relatively good quality of life up until the last few weeks of his life. He seemed happy enough in his own way even though he must have known the end was near whether it turned out to be he had a matter of days, weeks or years left. I have given at the end of this book a copy of the speech I wrote to be read out at his funeral. It was true that he loved life and lived it to the full. There is a HUGE difference between someone asking to have their suffering end and a person feeling it would be kinder to end suffering.

With that in mind, I can't help but feel those poems were written more for my sake than his. I didn't end up taking his life, HD and pneumonia did that, but I can't help feeling guilty all the same that a part of me felt my husband would be better off dead at times. "Be careful what you wish for" as the saying goes.

The final poem was written before my husband died. With HD, as with other so called terminal illnesses, there is often a case of 'anticipatory grief'. I was grieving a long time before my husband died and I am sure he grieved too. I would be very surprised if people reading this book, who are doing so because of HD being in their lives, are not also in the process of grieving. They might just not recognise is yet.

The Dyno Rod

Introduction

There is a hilarious episode in John Harding's book 'What we did on our holiday' where the son (Nick) is asked by the mother to deal with an extremely large stool in the lavatory pan. The stool had been deposited by the father who had Parkinson's disease. I did even write in my blog at one point about 'Pooh Stick' which was the affectionate name I gave a metal mop handle used to help unblock the toilet at times.

Whilst written in a light hearted way there is a serious side to my poem. Many infirm people get to a stage where constipation becomes chronic. Lack of exercise; inadequate diet; and lack of fluids do not help.

It's never a nice thing for any carer to have to deal with, and very embarrassing for the patient too, but like a number of the poems in this Section I thought it deserved a place as much as anything else. People can die of embarrassment if being embarrassed about basic bodily functions means they are not attended to. Constipation can have all sorts of ramifications on the system and, where the opposite to constipation applies, lack of attention to hygiene can lead to compromising skin tissue and pressure sores.

If the title 'What we did on our holiday' sounds familiar the book was adapted for television in 2006 and shown on ITV1. The character of Nick was played by a remarkable British actor. Fortunately for the actor the toilet scene was not included. The actor is remarkable not just in his acting skills but in his caring and charitable nature. Nick was played by none other than one Shane Richie, Patron of the HDA.

There was a time behind closed door,
When privacy was key,
But now discretions' in the past,
Where you depend on me.

I know what goes inside your mouth,
I feed you every day,
It must expand when it goes south,
Is all that I can say.

God knows how come you do not faint,
Considering the girth,
It's not so much you're passing stools,
It's more like giving birth!

The toilet pan is full again,
So 'Pooh stick' gives a prod,
Another stomach churning job,
Just call me Dyno Rod!

The Flow Chart

Introduction

When my husband reached the point he needed proper incontinence support we were assigned a nurse who specialised in that area. Ultimately we ended up deciding it was best to use what they call 'all in one' pads.

Like all aspects of HD... illness... life in general... good things can come out of bad. I never made a big thing about the little 'accidents' when they started happening. The poor love was embarrassed enough as it was and I always managed to make excuses or light of it for his sake and mine. However, it was one thing having to clear up in the home but quite another whilst out in public. Fortunately we always managed to avoid an accident in public but it wasn't easy at times.

My husband was very good at taking fluids normally but when incontinence became a problem he was naturally more nervous about taking drinks on board. I was also nervous about giving him too much fluid, especially if going out of the house. As you can imagine that had a knock on affect and, whilst my husband didn't get any urine infections, dehydration did have an effect on his body at times.

I mention in an article reproduced in Section 8 'Time for Change' my husband's penchant for asking what time his pad was changed and how many pads he had used. It was a bit annoying at the time but he went through a stage of associating pad changes with pleasing me.

Where I had expressed delight at soiling his pad after he went through a stage of retaining his water for a very long time, my husband then took it that I was very pleased every occasion he needed changing. He then wanted to keep count of how many times he had gone each day.

I used to keep charts anyway so it wasn't a big thing but I did have to buy inserts which could be removed and replaced easily so as not to waste a whole pad each time if there was only a tiny flow.

Using the double tabs on the side of the pad, I was able to open the front; remove the inserts (two night time sanitary pads side by side); clean my husband; replace with two new inserts; and then re-seal the all in one pad without ruining it.

For anyone using all in one pads with two different colours on the sticky side tabs they are different for a reason. The upper sticky can be pulled up leaving the lower sticky in place and not at risk of tearing the pad. The upper sticky can then be re-sealed. This results in less waste and also less hassle. I often wish there was a training camp for carers where we could get advice and training and pass on little tips to make life easier. I have just probably confused more than enlightened. Diagram anyone?

"Oops there's a puddle, it could be your cup?
Don't worry my love, I'll soon clean that up."
As I run to the cupboard to go find my mop,
He can't hide his embarrassment, head starts to drop.

I change him once more, and make light of the stain,
He is mortified now that it's happened again.
Once so smartly dressed he's now sadly resigned,
To wear track bottom trousers, fast exit designed.

Too soon comes the point where it can't be denied,
That it's best to wear pads, other methods now tried.
The catheter painful where tugging on skin,
And the mess even worse, where the tube won't stay in.

At least with the pads he can sit there for hours,
No worry of accidents, rushing for showers,
Now come to terms with it, he's drinking more,
His hydration better than ever before.

The ENT Theory

Introduction

In December 2009 I submitted an article through Triond which made it onto the 'HealthMad' site. At the time of writing this introduction that article has my highest rate of views. It suggests people out there are either clicking on it as they want to check whether the woman REALLY HAS just written an article about nasal passages and snot, or there are a lot of people who share my concern that such an important issue doesn't seem to get enough attention. Maybe they are desperately trying to find advice or fellow worriers?

By way of introduction to this poem I have reproduced the article below:

'The Importance of Nasal Care in Huntington's disease

This article raises a bit of a taboo. No one ever talks about cleaning out their own nose let alone that of someone else. However, the quality of life and health of a person is too important to shy away from just because we are embarrassed by the subject

The following observation is made in the hope that someone in the medical profession will either challenge my observations and prove me wrong, or take up on my theory here and look into what can be done about what could be an important factor in the quality of life for those with HD and other illnesses.

My husband was diagnosed in 2005 with HD. The diagnosis was forced when his symptoms were becoming a danger to himself and others. I had noticed the symptoms for at least 5 years prior to diagnosis.

Even before diagnosis his motor skills had become such that he could not easily hold a tissue in order to blow his nose properly. Even with the tissue held precariously to his nose it became clear to me his cognitive skills were such that he couldn't really remember how to blow. The result was he would never really have a totally clear nasal passage.

In 2006 my husband reached the point where I took over his personal hygiene and care. I made it one of my first quests to tackle a build up of mucus which, by now, had gone hard and seemed to block his nasal passages totally.

The use of the corner of a flannel with lots of warm water, lots of tissues, latex gloves and obviously a strong stomach came into it. Once cleared out his speech and appetite seemed improved.

I don't believe my husband is alone in not having the motor functions and mental capacity to manage his own nasal clearing yet I have never seen anything about carers paying attention to this area. It's true that nature has its own ways of trying to ensure the mucus is discharged such as sneezing but that's certainly not been effective enough for my husband.

I've noticed that nasal cleaning has never been mentioned by any of the Speech and Language Therapists. I did mention that I ensure a clean nose is always maintained to one therapist who seemed genuinely surprised it hadn't been thought of before.

It stands to reason that a blocked nose will cause discomfort on many levels. In terms of aspiration I suspect it is a contributory factor as, if the nose can't take in air while the mouth is occupied chewing and swallowing, the mouth will want to keep opening and breathing into the lungs taking everything with it.

I am also mindful of making sure my husband's airways are clear after he vomits. The projectile generally means some of the substance will pass out of the nose. Without attention to cleaning it means he will have foodstuffs also mixed with mucus. Not only dangerous but unpleasant when trying to breath. Again he does not have the wherewithal to blow his nose properly after.

I appreciate it's not an easy thing to ask people to do for others no matter how close they are to the person, I'm also aware the patient needs to place a lot of trust in the person caring for them to allow such an intimate act. However, is there scope for more awareness of the importance of even just checking on the health of nasal passages when instructing and informing carers from a speech, language and dietary perspective?'

"Just eat another mouthful dear,
You've hardly touched your meal",
He's bunged up now, can hardly breath,
Imagine how you'd feel!

He knows he doesn't feel that good,
And food tastes very bland,
It's not just where he struggles now,
With cutlery in hand.

He forces down another bit,
And struggles with a swallow,
But in the process gags again,
And vomit starts to follow.

The plate is pushed aside again,
He goes back to his bed;
Another night of lack of food,
His appetite now shed.

Yet if she were to think it through,
Although she can't be sure,
His blocked nose could be what it is?
Once cleared would he eat more?

The Tug of Love

Introduction

When I was a child I saw a film called 'Whatever happened to Baby Jane'. It was an old Hollywood film starring Bette Davis and Joan Crawford. It horrified me that the disabled sister was served a rat on a plate as a kind on mental torment and torture by the other sister who had become her carer. The film was a horror thriller, and the carer had gone quite mad for reasons way beyond being a carer I hasten to add, but I still wondered how anyone could be such a cruel and evil old cow to someone so vulnerable?

I'm not saying I have done anything as nasty myself but I would be lying if I didn't admit there were times I was driven to being what could easily be termed as cruel or spiteful. The extra tug on the arm when having difficulty in dressing; the delay in doing something where in all honesty it didn't have to wait but doing it on my own time and terms felt I had control over the situation.

Even threatening a nursing home if all else failed to try to get some sort of understanding that I had no alternative but do what I was doing at the time. The threat was often accompanied by crying where I didn't feel I could cope anymore and the tears themselves must have tormented my husband where he would have helped me if only he could. Anger, a nursing home (his ultimate fear) and a crying self pitying woman. I still feel self loathing and shame when I think about how cruel that was even though I was always at my lowest ebb by then.

Years ago I would never have dreamt I could publically admit such a thing but from reading Hugh Marriott and John Harding I realised I was not alone. In 'The Selfish Pig's Guide...' there is a chapter entitled 'Pushing them down the stairs'. The whole chapter tries to help carers understand why they feel that way and how to recognise the signs be it overtly physical or subtle.

John Harding's 'What we did on our holiday' describes the sheer frustration and desperation of the wife when her husband's head is lolling to one side. She cannot cope. Not just with the physical difficulties this makes but the emotional recognition that progression is now going beyond her ability to help him. As I have mentioned before... Whilst writing about Parkinson's disease it could just have easily been HD. I have been there...

Neither writer sets out to condone cruelty but, by even just acknowledging it happens, they helped me. I am sure along the way they have helped many others too, both carers and patients, or should that be victims, alike.

He's woken up in a foul mood again,
And resisting attempts to get dressed.
"WILL YOU GET YOUR ARM DOWN!",
She's screaming at him, at the end of her tether so stressed.

The arm gets yanked, and he gives out a yelp,
But she's far too angry to care;
No pity is given, he wasn't much help,
It's his own fault for leaving it there.

The dressing is over, he's now sat so quiet,
And he's looking all scared and forlorn;
The moment is gone and she see's what's she's done,
And she wishes she'd never been born.

Now his carer, his gaoler, and torturer too,
She feels she's an EVIL OLD COW!
She's driven by love, not hate for her man.
But that's not how it seems right now.

The Jealousy

Introduction

In the poem, 'The Touching Moments', I recall where my husband showed consideration and caring for me. Just over a year before my husband died he found a new love and I had to share him with her. Not another woman but an adorable toy cat which he cared for so touchingly.

I still have a video on my mobile phone which I was going to show his neurologist next time there was an appointment. Such was my husband's gentleness of stroking the cat, even with his clumsy hands through HD, that I didn't think anyone would believe me if they didn't see it for themselves.

The cat was a battery operated FurReal ® 'Lulu – Cuddlin Kitty'. My husband had always loved cats but we could no longer have a real one as his HD meant his hands were clumsy and both would get hurt.

I got the idea of the battery cat when researching 'Pat cats' as featured on a television programme about our feline friends. 'Pat cats' are used as therapy and are extremely tolerant. The good thing about the battery cat was I didn't have to hand her back after a session or clean up any mess. The bad thing was she cost a fortune in batteries as I needed to keep her on most of the day and even ended up buying five which I would sneakily swap over when running down on power etc.

Why did I keep her on and have so many? My husband's HD gave him a childlike innocence where his cognitive skills were being stripped from him one by one. Despite my initially mentioning she wasn't real when handing her over he chose to ignore that line and believe the cat was real. I couldn't break his heart by putting him right. If the cat went flat or broke down he would have thought she was dead

It got to the stage where I aided and abetted the lie by making sure she was responsive and I had answers. When he asked once why she couldn't walk like the other cats I told him she was disabled like him. I said she had been given bionic joints so she could be saved and come live with us. By sheer coincidence, a documentary on 'Bionic Pets' had been shown on the television. That seemed to satisfy his curiosity.

The cat was named "Ruby" by my husband and she played a part in helping him come back to me albeit so briefly on his final day. She's sitting a few feet away from me now, just the other side of the casket of his ashes. She and her fellow Rubys, apart from one which I gave to one of our carers (Flavia), keep me company now.

The final line of this poem seems harsh. I know my husband loved me in his own way but it still hurt that at the time he showed more affection for her than me in many ways. There are carers out there who are starved of affection. I was going to write a poem along those lines but didn't feel able to as I know how lucky I was to have my husband and it feels like a betrayal to write about him in that way now.

Although the dynamics of our relationship changed, in that I became his mother more than his wife, I am sure he still had feelings for me up until the day he died. Even now it feels he is here with me and Ruby, helping us carry on.

"She isn't real" she softly said,
When placed upon his knees.
The clumsy hands came down so slow,
Soft grasp instead of seize.

The look of love was clear to see,
A smile was breaking wide.
She walked away, emotions mixed,
The tears she'd need to hide.

The look of love, and hands so soft,
The tender touch and feel,
Were all for his new pussycat,
To him the cat was real.

"I love you cat" she heard him say,
It cut her like a knife.
This toy was loved above all else,
No feelings left for wife.

The Night Fighter

Introduction

This poem describes what it can be like to have someone you love tormented and tortured by HD even in their sleep.

Although the physical movements were contained when sitting upright in his armchair and then his wheelchair, for several years the disease struck my husband worst physically when in a lying position. Such was the extent of his thrashing out and Myoclonus (likened to the whole body hiccupping violently) he needed a special bed with four inflatable high sides strapped tightly to the bed itself to stop him banging his head and feet, breaking limbs, or even rising to the point of jumping/falling out of the bed!

He often cried out and whimpered. Sometimes he would claw at his own head as if trying to rip the illness out of himself. What must be have been going through his mind?

Ding-ding; Round One; its seconds out;
The punches start to rain.
No boxing ring or ropes in sight,
He's in his bed again.

The eyes are closed, he's fast asleep,
Yet body knows this not.
To stop the bruised and battered limbs,
His 'SafeSides'® form a cot.

And all the while, a noise he makes,
Like wounded dog in pain.
His brain tormenting during sleep,
His face contorts again.

As morning comes he quietens down,
And finally at ease.
A few short hours of peace and rest,
Have mercy on him PLEASE!

The Bedtime Prayer

Introduction

This poem was penned at around 2:30 in the morning after another night of tidying up after my husband had gone to bed. There was no point in going to bed myself. I was rarely able to settle immediately so usually got up after a while anyway.

Although I refer to 'cries of pain' in this poem as I had done so in the poem before, there was no way of telling whether physical pain was actually being felt by him. When I asked if he was "in pain" he always shook his head. However, I was not sure if he actually comprehended what pain was, or simply could not express he felt it. To my mind though, whether physical or mental pain applied I couldn't help but feel it for him.

Until the very final months of my husband's life, when the body jerks dampened down a bit, it was impossible for me to sleep. Not just his thrashing out in the bed where his limbs flailed but the noises he made. I was exhausted emotionally and physically most of the time. In fact... I found this on my Computer (PC) a week after I wrote it. Such was my auto pilot state of being I couldn't even remember writing it.

Several months after writing, towards the end when the sleep disturbance was lessened through his body probably being too weak to thrash about, I would still lay in bed listening for him in case he needed me. Then there was the checking on him constantly, scared he was not asleep, but dead. Much like a paranoid mother...

It's 2am and sleep can wait,
PC logged on, don't care it's late.
She catches up on missed TV,
It's downtime now, this times' for ME.

The headphones on as quiet needed,
His cries for help will go un-headed.
A wait of several minutes more,
The headphones placed upon the floor.

On hearing noise she makes a leap,
To enter room, he's fast asleep.
The help she heard were cries of pain,
His mind asleep but gone insane.

And now disturbed, she goes to bed,
And lies awake, his screams in head.
As morning comes, she'll fall asleep,
I lay me down, our souls to keep.

Cheating Life

Introduction

In 'The Night Fighter' I described how tortuous it is to have Huntington's haunt you even while your body should be at rest in sleep.

This poem describes the feeling of relief when the rest finally comes, for sufferer and carer. Maybe the ultimate relief would be kinder?

The above part of the Introduction and the poem below were written before my husband died. I do not regret penning this poem or including it. My husband is at peace now and even if tomorrow a cure were to be announced it would probably have been too late for him. We all have to die at some point (my only true comfort in all this). It felt like he was ready to go and I was ready to let him go.

He lays there still, his breath so deep,
His peace at last, they savour sleep.
She watches over, holds the moment,
He stops the twitching, stops the torment.

His mind at rest, or so it seems,
But who knows what, will haunt his dreams?
Her heart feels pain, new breath is taken,
Her wish not granted, he will awaken.

Another day, of his demise,
And life presents, its twisted prize.
For death is mercy, feels his wife,
She prays one night, he will cheat life

The Pillow Fight

Introduction

In my previous poems I tried to capture how hard it was watching someone deeply distressed by illness even in their sleep.

This poem builds on it to the point of potential euthanasia. However, it's not an easy thing to do under any circumstances.

He's twitching, contorting,
And stuck in his pain.
Not physical torture,
It's happening again.

His mind is convulsing,
His murmurs scream out,
The body is thrashing,
Stuck mind tries to shout.

The pillow picked up now,
Just inches from head.
With just one more push now,
She'll make sure he's dead.

But arms cannot lower,
Her heart is the brake,
She'll watch over him now,
She'll stay fast awake.

And morning will break now,
And she'll breathe relief.
Her day starts with life now,
Instead of with grief.

The Grief

Introduction

In 1969 Dr Elizabeth Kübler-Ross, a Swiss born American psychiatrist, wrote a best-selling book called 'On Death and Dying'. Dr Kübler-Ross dedicated her career to closely studying the emotional and psychological needs of the terminally ill. In her work she went on to describe five stages of grief.

Interpreted very loosely they cover:-

Denial: "This can't be happening to me!"

Anger: "Okay... It's happening... I didn't do anything wrong or deserve this so who do I blame for this?"

Bargaining: "Okay, you win... I accept it is happening but let's come to some arrangement here. If I promise to live a better life now and give up something will you just let me live to see another birthday?"

Depression: "I may as well give up. I've run out of answers. I can't do anything so why bother with anyone or anything?"

Acceptance: "We have all got to die one day. My time just happens to be sooner than others. I am ready, and I am at peace with what is coming".

Although the observations of Dr Kübler-Ross were based on people dying of cancer in hospital, her findings could easily be considered to apply to the phases of grief in many other circumstances of death and indeed life.

It's very sad that HD is referred to as a terminal disease. It takes many years normally from onset of being symptomatic to death itself. However, with there being no cure at present, telling someone they have tested positive, or even telling someone they are at risk, may have just as much of a devastating impact as telling someone they have a disease with a very short life expectancy.

And then there is the Anticipatory Grief element. The following has been taken from a Cruse Bereavement Care training brochure:

'What is anticipatory grief?

Lindermann (1944) first used the term.

Anticipatory grief as a concept is interpreted in different ways:

❖ *Relating to grief that occurs in preparation of impending death*

❖ *A journey towards the ultimate loss through a death, but is composed to adjusting to many losses, of the past, present and future.'*

Everyone deals with grief differently, be it after the actual death of a person or anticipatory grief. The following poem was written as a kind of duet. Both parties grieving for the same things but in different senses. It is ultimately about anticipatory grief. The person with HD himself grieving as much as the carer. The loss of self being acknowledged here.

I do miss and grieve for my husband but because of how the disease was, and how I feel it would be selfish to wish he were back here now, it feels wrong to mourn him in many ways. It's strange but it feels as though because of the anticipatory grief I have moved straight on to Stage five:

Acceptance:
"We have all got to die one day. *His* time just happened to be sooner than others. I am ready, as I have to believe *he* was, and I am at peace with what happened to *him*".

Will the other phases come back to hit me like a tonne of bricks? We shall have to wait and see...

Her to Him

I grieve for the man I used to know;
I grieve for the places we once used to go;
I grieve for the life we shared together;
I grieve for the wit from one so clever.

Him to Her

I grieve for the man I used to be;
I grieve for the places I'll never see;
I grieve for the walks held hand in hand;
I grieve for the wit I no longer command.

Her to Him

I grieve for the times, both good and bad;
I grieve for the intimacy we once had;
I grieve for the future we'll now never see;
I grieve for the loss of you and me.

Him to Her

I grieve for the memories once in my head;
I grieve for loss of you in my bed;
I grieve for loss of planning my life;
I grieve for the loss of you as my wife.

Together

The saddest part is it wasn't the dying;
That led to the grief and the sorrow and crying;
This grief has been growing in you and in me;
From the very first day that we heard of HD.

Section 8

The
Caring
Of
Angels

And as another Angel,
Collects their golden wings,
They leave behind their legacy,
For living human beings.

Introduction to Section 8

The Caring of Angels

I'm not sure who first coined the phrase 'HD Angel' when referring to those who have died in HD circles. The first time I heard the term was in connection with the loss of children having been struck by Juvenile HD. On the HDA Message Board we now often announce the death of a loved one as another HD Angel whatever their age. As you can imagine it is sadly all too often we hear the announcement.

By using the title 'The Caring of Angels' I wanted to give it two meanings. The first being that this Section shares stories about caring for our loved ones with HD, and the second from the viewpoint that I hope both Angels featured (My husband Steve and Myrna's daughter Rikki) are happy that their stories may help others. The Angels are caring for not only us but for strangers they will never meet.

The first story, 'Time to Change' has previously been mentioned under other poems. I included the article in this book to try demonstrating how ingenious we all have to be when it comes to HD and the irrationality of it all at times. I was feeling rather proud of myself at the time but the benefits where sadly short lived.

Some of my last posts before my husband died were desperate pleas for ideas on how to help my husband's neck from lolling to one side. In fact, the day before he died the Occupational Therapist visited to see if there was anything we could do. I remember saying to her on the way out that if Steve managed to pull through that stage it would only be delaying the inevitable but I had to try. Never give up trying...

The next three stories were featured within a blog I was writing and sending out on a Pay to View basis. I called the fundraiser 'Pimp My Blog' and the money went towards the HDA. Rikki's Story had been written several months before I was blogging but Myrna, the author, kindly let me use it as an appendix the week Rikki would have been 28. References to these stories are made in several of the poems.

The last entry is the speech I prepared for Steve's funeral. I have omitted some of the names where there is still the sad reality that his brother and sister don't want people knowing about HD in the family. My understanding is both are at risk untested as at time of writing and neither wishes to test. I may be stirring up a whole hornet's nest by putting this book in the public domain but I will take my chances with that

TIME To Change

Introduction

The following entry is taken from an article I submitted on a writers' site – Triond. I joined Triond when looking for ways to get my poems and writings in the public domain so that I could get feedback. Just like my Blog it helped to use writing as therapy and this particular article helped me polarise my thoughts on trying to always offset the bad side of HD against the good side.

YES... My husband infuriated me at times but it was the disease and not him and he gave me some wonderful challenges along the way. But... I'd like to think we made a pretty formidable team. I miss him very much now and still keep the clocks going. As I type this sentence it is 47 days, 20 hours and 17 minutes since he died.

Triond article:

'Clock Watching

Sometimes it helps to be devious when dealing with Huntington's disease. Here's how I used my husband's fixation with clocks to help him.

My husband has Huntington's disease (HD), formerly known as Huntington's Chorea. As anyone caring for someone with HD will probably recognise they can have a tendency to get fixated on things. One of my husband's key fixations is time. Not just everything has to be done at the exact same time each day but he has to have his clock within view.

The fixation thing can be infuriating as I actually have to take the clock off the wall and place it in front of him for every activity. I actually have three of the same clocks strategically placed around the home (he thinks they are the same one) but when I wheel him into the wet room to give him a shower he screams blue murder until I take the clock off the bedroom wall and place it in front of him to see. Wall clocks, fully tiled wet rooms and showers don't go well together therefore I can't keep one on the wall in there. I have to balance it on a bucket! Lately the fixation thing came in handy though.

My husband tends to slope to his left a lot. To help correct his posture we took delivery of a new specialist chair. Unfortunately the chair was not adjusted properly and, as a result, he not only ended up sloping even more to his left but his neck began to get crooked to the left! The chair has since been altered but the neck was still leaning to the side.

Whilst a neck brace could have been of help to your average person there was no way my husband would tolerate a neck brace. In fact... trying to get anyone with HD at mid-late stage progression (which my husband is) to do something they don't want to is fighting a losing battle. It then occurred to me. What if I were to use what HE wants to do?

Now this is going to sound tedious I know but trust me on this. It is a lot less tedious than living with someone whose head is lolling to one side, making their neck go to one side, making their shoulder slope, and in turn off-setting their whole body line and shifting their weight.

Over a week I placed Hubby's clocks from being in front of him over to his right hand side thus forcing him to move his head to the opposite side where it was sloping. He spends a good few hours in bed staring at a clock from his pillow. He likes to bark orders at me for his drink at 10 in the morning and get up at 11 and note in his mind at what time he used his incontinence pants (DON'T ASK).

With Hubby needing to stretch his neck over to the other side he gradually managed to strengthen his neck and now his alignment is MUCH better! Now all I need to do is work out how to sneak in and adjust all three atomic clocks so that I can get an extra hour sleep. Damn those atomic clocks, they keep resetting themselves. Grrrrrrrr

"One scoop of patronisation or two?"

Introduction

The following was written as part of my fundraising blog exercise 'Pimp my Blog'. I have reproduced the article where I referred to it in the poem 'The Wheelchair'.

With HD many patients need a lot of gentle persuasion to do things as they do not like change. In this example it took a lot of bravery for my husband to accept using the wheelchair for the first time and we were set back quite a way by someone being thoughtless.

We never returned to the restaurant again!

Saturday 14th June 2008

Hubs had wanted to get up early today to get his hair cut and go to the 'Italian' Place. The place he means is actually run by a Turkish family I think but I'm happy to call it Italian as I think Hubs counts any place that serves lovely ice cream as Italian.

We used to go there regularly on a Saturday afternoon when we first came to Greenwich last year. We stopped when the footy season started as Hubs likes his footy on a Saturday and doesn't consider he can go to the place any other day [than a Saturday] so as he can't do both on one day...

It's a five minute walk from here to the hairdressers for me but half an hour for Hubs. When you add another 15 minute walk from the hairdressers to the restaurant for him I was concerned whether he would be too tired so I asked him outright if he would be alright using the wheelchair? To my surprise Hubs said "Okay".

It was the first time I had actually got him to sit in the thing and I'd already been worried about how his feet would cope as there were no straps to hold them onto the foot plates. Needless to say within a few minutes of being pushed his feet were on the floor and I kept having to stop to reposition them and just pushing the thing on a flat area was difficult. I should add that we were having problems even before we'd left the block as the bloody communal doors are fire doors and so heavy.

Hubs is now over 10 stone and as much as the Enshakes and Creatine are saving his life it's making mine a problem. With his being 2 stone heavier than he was this time last year it was a nightmare trying to tilt the chair to manage kerbs. Even with the slope for chairs there is usually some need for tilting.

With the road works outside The Mitre Pub it meant an impossible task of cutting across the road halfway down. I was relieved when a bloke offered to help and between us we managed to get Hubs back on the pavement. What with my being so small, and I think he heard me saying to Hubs "You'll have to get out of the chair a moment" it's not surprising he felt obliged to help.

When we got to the hairdressers Hubs got out of the chair and I folded it so as not to be a nuisance in such a small shop. The Barber was great with him this time and he managed to get in and out of the barber chair without damaging himself and giving everyone a heart attack.

When we left he was happy to get back into the wheelchair and have me push him to the restaurant. He got out of it to walk into the place but it was awkward trying to get him up the step; handle a heavy folded chair, and also the seat pad which has to come out in order for the damn thing to fold. Seeing my struggle the proprietor came over and took the chair whilst I saw to Hubs.

I had my usual (a glass of wine) whilst I fed Hubs a huge banana split which comes with lots of fruit and two flavours of ice cream and strawberry or chocolate sauce and cream. He devoured it as ever with an orange juice and latte after, plus a sip of my desert (a large port)! He was a full and happy bunny apart from being annoyed with me that I'd forgotten to bring along his afternoon cod liver oil capsule. He has it with orange juice you see... I say he was a happy bunny but that didn't last for either of us. It didn't even last pass paying the bill. Not that the bill was the problem. The place serves excellent food and drink and the price is excellent value. The thing was this...

Like I mentioned earlier we had been going to the place regularly last year. The guys there recognised us instantly and even asked where we'd been all this time so I said we'd been busy as you do. In the past they've always helped pull the table out for Hubs and known I feed him etc, but we all had chats about the area and passed the time of day quite normally. I can only assume it was the addition of the wheelchair that made the proprietor treat Hubs like some deaf and dumb mute this time!

When he handed us the bill he asked me "what is this man to you? Are you his friend, are you related?" I answered he was "My Husband". He then asked

"How long you two been together?" "Was he like this when you met him?" I tried my best not to look too stunned and told him we are celebrating our 20th wedding anniversary this year and that Hubs had HD and it's only these last few years he's been ill etc but I was choked the guy suddenly felt he needed to bypass Hubs and address me in such a way. I was mortified for Hubs who just sat there having to listen to it!

I couldn't get out of the place quick enough and knew Hubs was probably mortified and embarrassed at the guy helping us with the chair again. Needless to say the ride home was a lot quicker and quieter. I knew all the landmark work we had done that day had now been undone by the thoughtless actions of someone meaning well. What was meant to be a special treat for Hubs and a trial of the chair would probably mean he wouldn't want to get back in the thing again and I'm not sure if Hubs will want to go back there again although I will ask in a few weeks time and see what his reaction is.

The rest of the day was quiet and the chair was put in my bedroom out of sight again. I had hoped to brooch the subject of taking it to Llandudno with us the following week but knew it wasn't very practical anyway. Now, on an emotional side, I couldn't bear it if the staff at Hub's favourite hotel started treating him the way the restaurant had. It was bad enough last time when one of the porters had to help me get him out of the bath where he fell in (long story involving the toilet – another treat in store for readers on another day when I am feeling more up to sharing the delights of 'Pooh Sticks')

Breaking Point

'God grant me the serenity to accept the things I cannot change,
The courage to change the things that I can,
and the wisdom to know the difference'

(Rienhold Niebhur)

Introduction

I wrote the following as part of another writing exercise I was doing but I inserted it as an appendix to my blog to illustrate something. I got a fair bit of feedback from people who had obviously been thinking of therapy for some time but were unsure as to whether they would benefit.

It worked for me at that particular stage in my life. That doesn't say it would always work for others, and for some who could benefit I'm aware the options to take advantage of it are sadly just not there.

There came a time later on when I really needed to look into Therapy again but I didn't have the flexibility at that time which was needed to attend the sessions (run by the mental health service 'mind'). A catch twenty two situation... I was feeling suicidal where I felt trapped at home being a carer but I couldn't do anything about it as I was trapped at home being a carer. Nonetheless, I thought I would insert this episode to highlight I am no saint and we all need help from time to time.

By way of background we were living in Erith in Kent in a one bedroom flat. I was sleeping on the floor by the bed, where it was impossible to share the bed with my husband's movements during the night, yet I needed to be in the same room lest he fall out of the bed.

We had a nuisance neighbour who played the same record – YES the SAME one record – again and again at full volume for hours on end. We had gangs of youths riding up and down our cul de sac every weekend on noisy quad bikes. I had moved to a more local office (Bexleyheath Police Station) to make things easier at home only to be rapidly promoted to a very pressurised job as Finance and Resource Manager on the basis I would have lots of support, only to have my boss suddenly go off on sick leave for several months. To cap it all, a few weeks into the job, the London Seven July bombings occurred making my job as Finance and Resource Manager covering three Metropolitan Police Stations a complete nightmare.

My husband's needs were becoming more and more severe yet I was spending more time apart from him at work than ever (part the job and part my wanting to get away from the struggle at home); and I was drinking far too much for my own good. The weekend I wrote about was a turning point. The straw that broke the camel's back...

The Therapy

With the strain of coping with Steve, the backlash of the London bombings of 7/7 on my job, the frustration of living in Frobisher with Mr Nutter and his loud music downstairs, and Erith's answer to mini Brand's Hatch come Isle of Man Bike Rally on my cul de sac, I took it upon myself to book Steve and I for a weekend at one of our favourite hotels from years gone by. They say you should never return and how true that is.

Years ago we had booked Christmas at a hotel in Malden in Essex. The whole experience was so peaceful and still fun as the owners went that extra mile to make all their guests have a wonderful Christmas, with just the right mix of festivities for those seeking company and space for those wanting to get away from it all. Steve and I often reminisced about our time there so I thought it would be ideal to go back and get away from all the noise and other issues.

By now I was working virtually ten hours a day seven days a week and, because of Steve, I would be getting in at seven in the morning and sometimes going back at midnight once I had been home to make sure he was settled. It was no life and I was surviving on adrenalin and alcohol.

I knew that if I didn't get away from home I would be tempted to go into work and I owed it to Steve as well as myself to make time for us. When we arrived at Perville Station the signs were already beginning to look ominous. The cab we had pre-booked turned up late and nearly run over my foot when the idiot driver tried to shoot off whilst I was still settling Steve in the car.

The hotel allocated us a room on the top floor which is not ideal for Steve but they didn't have anything else. Apart from the stairs there was also another thing that filled my heart with dread the moment we stepped inside our room. The last time we had stayed we were given a lovely room in the yard of converted stables. This time we were smack on the side of the main building, just off the main road, and within about six yards of the village church. You could see the church bell tower from the window and as if that weren't enough its bell loudly chimed on the quarter hour and fully on the hour.

We made it down for dinner and I was determined not to be annoyed but I was already getting stressed out. After a few drinks and a lovely meal I relaxed a little but the bells ringing early on the Saturday morning made me tense again. After breakfast I dragged Steve out along the high street to get some magazines, a few treats, and bought half of Boots in terms of scented bath oils, body rub, and soaps etc.

On the way back we stopped off in a coffee shop for lunch and then I began to realise the devil himself was out to get me. Before I could get comfortable in my chair the noise of car horns and bikes revving up sent deafening vibrations throughout the café. I should have realised there was an unusually large mass on the pavements before but I had to ask the waitress.

Sure enough, it was a festival weekend with biker parade and brass bands with carnival floats etc. I literally started shaking with rage when I heard all the noise and my already frayed nerves went into shock syndrome.

We got back to the room but could still hear the Parade. Fortunately the bathroom was able to mute the sound a bit and I was determined to have my relaxation time. I spent an hour in the bath in the dark with the aromatherapy sensations and when my time was up I went into the bedroom and lay on the bed relaxed. The carnival was over and I got a whole hour sleep before it was time for Steve to get me up to get ready for dinner.

* *

When Steve woke me I felt like a new woman. Even the bells from the church seemed to be muffled and I was ready to enjoy the hotel's excellent cuisine with a glass or three of their red wine. I hadn't taken out my frustrations too badly on Steve yet and that, for me, was a good sign. After all, this was about him as much as me. He needed to be shown I still cared and had his welfare at heart too.

We dressed for dinner and both looked very presentable. My makeup was immaculate and I was able to put on my favourite things. We had already agreed to go into the annexed pub across the yard for a pre-dinner drink, as we loved the quaintness of it. When we walked in the rugby was on the telly and three guys were at the bar talking sport. Steve and I grabbed a table and I went to the bar to get him a pint of lager and my glass of Merlot. I think I must have had all of two sips before it happened.

As a child and teenager I used to watch Saturday night telly with my family and laugh along with the next person at the antics of the comedian Jack

Douglas. He would be doing his sketch and then suddenly his arm or leg would jerk out with no warning and take him by surprise with comedic effect shouting "phweeey" as he looked bemused at what happened.

Unbeknown to me at the time, his twitching was later compared to taking the proverbial out of Huntington's sufferers. I have no idea whether Jack Douglas had ever seen anyone with HD though. Steve has those moments albeit without the cry. They devastate him when in public and in one such moment he managed to experience an involuntary full shock of the arm sending his whole pint over me.

It wasn't on purpose, I know that, but at the time all I could think about was how all my effort to relax and look good had gone to waste and how the barman would have thought he was a drunk or that we had been fighting.

* *

One of my survival techniques is gritting my teeth. I calmly got up from my chair drenched in lager and walked over to the bar where the guys were watching me and trying not to laugh. With my hair, face and clothing dripping lager I asked for a cloth to wipe up the mess whilst the barman said he would clear it and was already pouring another pint for Steve obviously having already taken in Steve was not quite all there and it wasn't his fault.

In my sheer anger and embarrassment I walked over to Steve, placed his new pint before him and said we should drink up, as I wanted to go back to our room. He must have got about four sips through before I gulped down my red wine, still standing from not wanting to sit on the wet chair. At that stage I said I was going back to the room and he should stay there. I stormed back to the room and I still don't know what made me leave the door open but, quite frankly, I had every intention of packing my bag and leaving Steve that night.

Steve must have sensed the serious level of my state as he somehow managed to manoeuvre his way out of the pub, across the courtyard, up the stairs and into our room. He is not totally disabled as I have said before but believe me when I say it was hard for him to do that on his own.

When he entered the room he saw me packing the case and sat on the bed pleading with me not to leave him. By now I was enraged and told him I couldn't go on with the way things were and I wanted to kill myself. I wrote down his mother's number for him to call and make sure she picked him up the next day but I was seriously going to walk off that night and make my way back home alone via the off-licence and pop a few pills.

I allowed myself to meet Steve in the eye and saw his true vulnerability. I felt akin to a mother and realised I couldn't bring myself to abandon him. As much as I was feeling sorry for myself it wasn't fair to take it out on him.

I had to vent my frustration somehow and I raised my hand. It was either going to be slapping and beating Steve or turned on myself. I proceeded to slap my head and face like a mad woman. It scared Steve even more but when I finished I felt cleansed and calmly put on fresh clothes over my still beer drenched body and took Steve down to dinner as though nothing had happened. When I retired to bed that night, after a shower, I knew I had reached a dangerous place and needed help.

* *

When we woke the next morning nothing was said about the night before but the feeling of self-disgust still filled me. We had breakfast and got ready for our journey home but I knew I had come very close to leaving Steve, killing myself, or killing him. With my having been taken out of the work arena at the time of trauma I couldn't blame it all on my job. I therefore knew I would have to do something fast to stop myself from killing one of us.

The previous day I had bought some magazines that I had foolishly expected to read during a relaxing afternoon and evening. On the train home I picked up one of the mags and soon found myself reading an article on Stress. Obviously I read it expecting to think the authors wouldn't know what stress was if they were hit in the face with it by a bat! I did, however, get drawn to the help strap line. The article impressed me with its serious and knowledgeable take on the subject and gave a number of contact points including the website for the British Association for Counselling and Psychotherapy.

When I arrived home I looked up their website and managed to trace a counsellor very near to my work in Albion Road, Bexleyheath. I sent off an e-mail asking to be contacted for an appointment and the guy telephoned me the next day offering me a slot that week. I could even fit it into my lunch hour thus not interfering with anything else. The guy was named Michael Barratt and I probably owe him my life if truth were told.

During our first session he sat and listened to me explaining why I felt I needed to refer myself. He asked questions at the right moments but most of all he just offered me a box of tissues and let me cry and pour my heart out. After about forty minutes he reassured me I was entitled to feel sorry for myself and I had every right to seek help. My doing that confirmed I was coping more than could be expected of someone with so many demands on them and he would be there for me as a sounding board.

I had seriously considered I was going under and wondered if going to a therapist would lead me to being referred to a doctor and then some medication which had scared the shit out of me. The last thing Steve and I needed was for me to be given tranquilisers, or worse of all taken away from him. I was so relieved Michael was able to reassure me that I was not mad. I was also worried any forced medical intervention would need to be notified to my boss at the Police Station.

We went on to have two further sessions and by then I was handling my incident of self- loathing better. It was agreed I would contact Michael again if I needed any more help but in essence I had got through the pressure cooker stage and was even learning to turn the gas down to below simmering.

I will never be able to turn the gas out completely. I wouldn't be human if I could do that given all the stuff chucked at me to cope with. Besides.... I'm one of those people who need a level of stress to feel alive. And god knows if there's potential for stressful situations I always seem to be drawn towards them.

Rikki's Story

Introduction

The following is reproduced by kind permission of Myrna Lyman. It is the text of a talk given by Myrna at an HDA Conference.

In Myrna's talk she explained what it was like to have a daughter who suffered from Juvenile Huntington's Disease, and how difficult it was at times especially when those who are meant to help did not even recognise that JHD existed!

Myrna writes not just of how hard things could be but also how privileged she was to have had Rikki in her life and how special Rikki was. Rikki died in 2007 aged just twenty seven.

I referred to this speech in my poem 'The Tooth Fairy'. Even before reading this I was aware of my husband's reluctance to have a PEG fitted when the time would come. The decision would always have been Steve's own decision but this story helped me in many ways. Not just enlightening me on things that might occur but in coming to terms with his feelings. It also gave me strength in those last few months and days when, like Myrna with Rikki, I knew the end was coming.

I am indebted to Myrna, as are many people, for having the courage to share her story.

Rikki's Story

By Rikki's mother – Myrna Lyman

My daughter Rikki lived with juvenile Huntington's disease for almost 14 years and it was only in her last year that I learned many new things from reading and talking to other family members who live with Huntington's disease via forums on the Internet while I was searching for answers since Rikki had taken a turn for the worst.

Before that, we just lived with HD as best we could. It would have been nice to have the support and understanding from other families who live with it during the years that I needed it. I found that the best way to cope was to concentrate on trying to make Rikki's life happy for her and creating wonderful memories for us all to treasure. We'd been told there was no hope and no cure, so to focus on creating extra happiness was the best we could do.

If I was to have any regrets, it would be that I didn't search the Internet sooner for much valued information which is in abundance on the HDAC Lighthouse, HDA and other forums where people get together to share their knowledge and experiences.

As well as finding info and sharing experiences, living with HD can be very lonely in respect of other people just 'not getting it'. Joining the forums helps to alleviate that loneliness. Knowing little about HD and being happy to bury my head in the sand, rather than go out and look for more information than I already knew, was something that stayed with me until Rikki took ill in February last year. In my mind it was terminal, what more did I need to know?

There have been many pitfalls along the way over those 14 years, some of which I believe could probably have been avoided or improved had I known there were better choices I could have made. I can't speak highly enough of the information and help that is available when you look for it.

* *

I first heard of Huntington's disease when I met Rikki's dad in 1979. I was 18. He was 20. He told me that his dad had died from it and that it was a mental illness. I accepted just that, he didn't elaborate and I didn't ask. Unfortunately his behaviour was one I couldn't accept nor understand, so we parted. I had no idea that he was showing early signs of HD until many, many years later. Soon after we parted, I discovered I was expecting Rikki.

When she was 5 years old, I was told that her dad had been diagnosed with Huntington's disease. My informer told me that it was hereditary and that Rikki had a 50% risk of developing it too. An appointment was arranged for me to see a specialist at our general hospital. He told me that no-one under the age of 40 developed HD and that most were much older, usually around the age of 60. He also said that children didn't develop it.

To be fair about what he did know, he advised me to have Rikki sterilised as soon as she began her periods....to prevent HD from being passed on to any children she might have. I was disappointed that he didn't take the time to explain anything more to me but I had no idea what to ask him. I've come to realise that not only then, but even recently, many doctors know very little about Huntington's disease and even less about the Juvenile form.

My biggest worry after the appointment was whether or not I should stop Rikki from having children, at an age when she wouldn't be quite old enough to decide for herself. After much thought, I came to the conclusion that I couldn't take that right away from her and anyway her children would be grown up before she'd develop it. I knew that no matter what she had to face, as a family, we would be there for her and for her children.

Worry over, we got back on with our lives as normal and mostly put HD to the back of our minds for the next few years. Now I know so much more about Huntington's, I am grateful that having children never became an option for Rik.

Rikki began changes which I really became aware of when she was 13. Though she'd had behaviour issue's that I can pinpoint back to the age of 8 or 9 for sure and even some way back to when she was a baby, I just put them down to her various ages and her personality. What I could see now though was different though difficult to explain.

I asked close family and friends if they could see something different about her, but no-one could. So I was just left to wonder...could I or couldn't I? At that time, it was small glimpses and not anything I could be specific about.

After a while, I began to suspect she was drinking alcohol or taking drugs, but those explanations didn't make sense considering she was rarely ever alone without me or one of her sisters. It didn't stop me from asking her though. The shocked look on her face was all the answer I needed to know that she wasn't.

One night a few weeks later, as I was drifting off to sleep and as weird as I know it sounds...a voice... might even have been a thought, although I hadn't been thinking about it...very clearly said...Rikki has Huntington's disease.

My eyes flew open and I knew she had it as sure as I know my own name...I had no doubts from then on. The next day I called Oxford and we were given an appointment with a neurologist in Northampton.

After talking to us and doing various balance type tests the neurologist said, "Rikki is not showing any signs of HD whatsoever. HD isn't something you should wish on your child". She told me not to be paranoid.

I'll never forget it. I was so shocked. I wanted to protest, but no words would come out of my mouth. I left the office in tears, but after a minute or two, I brushed them away because I knew she was wrong. I could see where she was coming from...if I struggled to explain it and others couldn't see it, then how could I expect her to?

Fortunately she did think to write to Rik's school and they replied saying they had seen a decline in her work as well as bad attitude toward her peers. We had one more meeting then the test was arranged.

This all began with the call in October 1995 and by February 96 it was confirmed that Rik did have Juvenile Huntington's Disease. I do hope that the neurologist has been more careful since with her choice of words when meeting other parents who suspect their child has HD. She did apologise to me after the result came back.

The evening before the test result, I brought home a puppy....something the girls had been asking for a long while. Charlie helped the girls to be distracted from those dreaded results in the following days and to continue the distraction tactic; we began to fund raise to take Rikki to Disney world in Florida.

I also liked the idea that our local Evening Telegraph would do an article about our reasons for fundraising and that this would explain to the people in our town just why Rikki was the way she was. I hoped it would help her school friends to accept her more easily....and it did!

I worked in a pub at the time and many people were willing to help us. Everyone rallied around and many events were set up to help raise the money and within just a few weeks, we had as much as we needed for all of us to go to Florida as a family.

It was such a busy time with attending these events and planning the holiday that we didn't have too much time to dwell on the whole meaning of having HD in our lives until after the coming back from Disney World.

I began to worry how I would keep working and care for Rikki too. I decided it would be good to run a pub of my own, - so that I could earn as well as spend time with the girls. It was hard work, but we had lots of fun doing it....probably not the best way to bring kids up, but for us it worked well for the time that we did it.

We were so surrounded by people and fun, that we didn't have time to dwell on any sadness, but as all things do, it had to come to an end when it became clear that Rikki was no longer taking care of herself. So we came out of the pub trade and I became Rik's full time carer. By now Rikki was 19.

For the first 10 ish years, I drank a lot to mask my feelings and to keep me on an 'up'. I was really scared of becoming depressed and not being able to cope and felt that alcohol helped me to cope better. When in actual fact it really was only a temporary mask.

* *

Once life settled down after Rik's diagnosis, I saw less and less of family and friends who had been a part of my life for so long. They just drifted away. Was that natural and would it have happened anyway? Or was it because of HD and its effects on us all. I don't suppose I'll ever really know or that it even matters now, but it certainly did to me then.

I just didn't have the time, energy or enthusiasm to be chasing friendships and putting in the effort that's required to keep them going so I had no choice but to accept my new circumstances and put up with the feeling of abandonment.

I found that pretty tough considering before HD, my house was the kind that was always busy...the door knocking, the phone ringing and people in and out all day all which added to the bedlam that I loved.

My days became in the most part, where it was just Rik and I when the rest of the family were out at work or school. I think we both found that kind of quiet a bit too tough for a while. On a couple of occasions, I tried going out to work, leaving Rik alone for a couple of hours a day. She was still fairly capable at that point.

One day her step dad, Joe, came home just in time to find some young lad bringing Rikki into the house. When questioned, he said he was helping her back from the shop. Rikki told us that she didn't know him and had only briefly met him once in a pub.

The thought of what could have happened scared me into giving up work there and then. So to keep myself busy in the years ahead, I became a decorator- holic. That's a different tale but it kept me busy inside my home for several years... while Rikki slowly declined.

* *

One of the biggest pitfalls I found from living with Huntington's is ignorance of the disease....other peoples as well as my own. I can't count how many times in the early days that people would make off hand comments about what it was that Rik was 'on' to make her as she was, or how many people outwardly laughed and mimicked her movements, made hurtful comments or just blatantly stared at her.

I can't count the many times I got cross with Rik for her behaviour in the early days....for her unreasonable jealousies when a sister had a birthday for instance or if I bought one of them a much needed item, such as school uniform.

There were the times when she would completely wreck the house from top to bottom in her angers because I couldn't afford to give her even more money or for some other seemingly trivial reason.

The stress that Rik must have felt, as well as the stress it put on us all individually was tough to bear at times. My ignorance in that was I didn't know there were certain medications that could have helped with those behaviours.

No one told us that certain symptoms were treatable and of course because I'd been told there was no hope or cure it just didn't occur to me. But, to be fair to anyone who could have told me, I always had to put on a face and I never told many people just how things really were. I always said we were coping and we were...just sometimes it was difficult.

I tried to tell one or two people how it really was during Rik's bad times, but it was easy to see that people thought I was exaggerating. They just didn't get that a person of Rikki's age could make such child like unreasonable demands or have such extreme tempers for no real reason.

They didn't get the obsessions or why she would use certain words repetitively. Nor did I for the longest time and there were times that my frustrations were apparent. I put a lot of Rikki's unreasonable behaviours down to her feelings of being told she had a terminal illness and tried to make allowances for her reasoning, but eventually I came to realise that it had to be something that HD was doing to her because she wasn't growing up and becoming mature in her thinking or reasoning.

Once I taught myself to handle her differently I was able to show more patience with her bad times.

* *

There was a time when Rikki's feet were turning purple so we went to see a specialist at the hospital who asked Rikki if she smoked. She did...10 a day. He looked at her and said you'd better stop or we'll have to amputate your legs...then he walked out, leaving me worried sick. Has anyone ever tried to tell a person with HD and extreme tempers that they have to stop smoking?? It didn't work!

The next visit we had with him, he brought the subject of smoking up again but this time he was angry with me because I was the one who bought Rikki's cigarettes for her because she couldn't. I tried to explain to him why I did, but he wouldn't listen and didn't want to know my reasons. In fact, he reported me to social services for abusing Rikki due to the cigarette burn on her finger and at our next review meeting the subject was brought up.

Little did he know that not only could I not stop her from smoking but trying to get her to put a fag out while there was still a bit of white on it, or to use a cigarette holder, was like trying to do the impossible?

Fortunately our HDA Regional Care Adviser was there at that review and she understood how you cannot force a person with HD to stop smoking. She wrote to him and told him and that thankfully was the last of that. I never did find out why Rikki's feet had turned the colour they had. Though they did eventually return back to normal. I just assume it was more to do with HD twisting them than it was to do with smoking.

* *

During the years we had various carers in to help. Some good... some not so good... and only one that stayed the distance. One of the difficulties of ever changing carers was training them to get used to Rik.

They needed to learn how to feel confident when helping her to walk and she needed to feel confident in their help or she would shake uncontrollably. They needed to understand her gestures and altered speech. They need to be patient and allow Rik to go at her own speed, which was very slow.

It took a while before I would feel confident enough to allow them to be on their own with her. And often it seemed that no sooner were we feeling confident, the carer would move on and we'd have to start all over again.

There was one new carer who on her first visit was happy to spend most of her time telling me about her marital problems. In between her words she would stand up to look at herself in the mirror. Of course I soon sussed her to be quite an odd lady, to say the least.

After she asked Rik a question, instead of being patient while Rikki struggled to reply, she said to her "come on Rikki, spit your words out". As you can imagine, it put Rik off what she wanted to say. And my temper began to bubble.

And then during feeding her she said to her "come on; open your mouth before your food goes cold" whilst pushing Rikki's dinner into her own mouth. I was mortified and furious with her. She had no interest in Rikki or her needs and no idea of what is was to be a carer for someone like Rik. Needless to say, I didn't allow her to return. Another carer came solely to help Rik to enjoy a social life. The intention was that Rik had some girlie time with someone other than family members...a break from us all.

We had a lovely girl who knew all about caring because she helped out with her grandma. She seemed pretty good, until a few weeks later when I went along to Rikki's local, just to have the landlady ask me why I allowed someone to bring Rik out who abandoned her while she socialised with others and got herself drunk, then drove Rik home.

Of course, not all carers were that bad. Mostly they just didn't stay very long which meant I spent a lot of time training people up and neither Rik nor I were getting the time out that having carers was meant to give us.

Eventually, I gave up and took on no more outside carers during the last couple of years...until the very end. If it hadn't have been from the loving care of Rikki's sisters, maybe I couldn't have carried out my promise to Rik to always keep her at home. They were great and did what they could when they could, when I needed them to. I don't know what I would have done without Carly the youngest, most of all... after Sarah and Beccy left home.

From the age of 6, she fell in with what needed to be done for Rikki and by the age of 11 she would toilet her, shower her and deal with many things that girls of that age really shouldn't have to. There was nothing that Carly wouldn't or didn't do for Rik. I said to her once. "Car, you shouldn't be doing these things for Rik and she looked at me surprised and said why? We're a family...we are all in it together" How sweet!

When we were in the pub, Sarah had already left home so Beccy took on the big sister roles ensuring that when I was working her sisters were fed and had clean clothes to wear. During Rikki's last months Sarah gave up her fairly new life in Manchester to move back to be close by. She started work for the care company that had been allocated to Rik so that she could help to give Rikki the best care, knowing how worried I was at having carers back in the house when they didn't know or understand Rik.

* *

One of the things I wish I'd known about, which I discovered after finding info on the net last year, is the extreme importance of dental care. Rikki's teeth were brushed daily as is the norm, but because of the difficulty she had in not being able to open her mouth, it was difficult to clean them properly and for the same reason, she hadn't seen a dentist in years.

Though I could see she had problems with her gums, I didn't take her to a dentist because I couldn't see what they would do for her if she was unable to open her mouth wide enough; and as I thought that every year would be Rikki's last, never understanding how much worse was to come, I never took the time to find out just what a dentist could do for her.

I don't suppose it helped me to make a sure decision because Rikki rarely seemed to feel pain either and she never complained or indicated she had problems...yet another downside to HD. For those reasons, I ignored her dental needs, much to my regret.

Last February, Rikki couldn't open her mouth to eat or drink. Overnight, her jaw clenched tightly shut. It took me 2 hours to get a couple of ounces of water into her via a gap in her teeth with a baby's medicine syringe.

I realised that she wouldn't be with us an awful lot longer if she couldn't get the nutrients her body needed and though I had tried to prepare myself for this day, I wasn't at all ready. The thought scared me so much that I was willing to go against Rikki's original wish of not having her life prolonged.

I made calls to arrange for her to have a PEG feed fitted. The first appointment we could get was in April for an assessment. I didn't believe she would be alive by then if she stayed as she was. The next day, it was obvious she was quite ill. We called the doctor in who sent her straight to hospital.

Once she was there it was arranged to have Rikki fitted with a PEG feed as soon as possible. I was relieved, even though the first dietician who assessed Rik said that she didn't need to be pegged as she could still swallow.

Hindsight is a wonderful thing isn't it? I look back now and feel very sure that the sudden over night jaw clenching was to do with dental problems. But at the time, I only saw what was in front of me...that Rikki could no longer eat or drink.

After Rik had been PEG fed we noticed a swelling on the side of her face...a sure sign she had an abscess. Rik was put on antibiotics and the swelling went down. I wish I could give an explanation as to what was going on with Rikki and why after that first spell in hospital.

All I can do is tell you that it's my conviction that medications she had been put on while in there were much to blame for a lot of unnecessary distress … and later something to do with the PEG feed somehow. That and the fact that we didn't know that there was dental problems to start with.

Suddenly Rikki began having severe movements…something she had never experienced before. Then she complained of being in pain. Then the throwing up several times a day began. It was so distressing for her and for me. The poor girl hardly had a moment's peace for the first 4 months. And many a night she was unable to sleep.

After months of searching, reading and talking to various people who live with HD, I was told by a Canadian pharmacist that the two meds she was on were reacting on the GABA receptors.

From that night I separated those meds and for the first time in 4 months for a whole weekend, Rikki's body stayed still and restful and I fully believed that if it wasn't for staff at the respite centre where she had stayed for a week and who made the unwanted decision to stop giving her food or drink against my wishes, Rik would have been pretty much back to her old self.

Sadly though, peace for her was short lived…due I'm sure to the medications as by now she had a cold and so a cold remedy was added to the meds she was already taking. Rikki's body began flinging itself all over the place again.

As it was she had lost the ability to swallow at all due to being out of practice for a week and by now fully depended on her Peg feed to sustain her. Due to the amount she was vomiting which continued to increase…Rikki was still losing weight and I could see we were still losing Rikki.

During this period of time we had the doctors out on an almost daily basis and she went back into hospital another 4 or 5 times. Sadly no-one at all had any idea of why there was a sudden yet devastating change for Rik. No-one was able to even come close to realising why.

To be honest, I was convinced back then that Rik's change was due to dental reasons in the first place…yet somehow things got out of hand when the meds were introduced… Peg feeding, aside…I'm as convinced now as I was when I first realised Rik had HD.

I absolutely regretted asking for the PEG feed to be fitted and wanted it removed to allow her to go naturally. I couldn't bear to see her suffer as she was and not one doctor or specialist knew what to do to help her.

I spoke to my GP and told him my feelings. Only it wasn't that simple. I wasn't allowed to remove the peg feed, and before anyone could make any decisions a lot had to be looked into.

* *

The palliative care team were sent in to help us and Rikki was put on morphine for the pain. It didn't take them long to see that even with the morphine, once her body adjusted to the dose, she was in pain again or for them to see that no sooner was she fed, she would bring it all back up again. In just a short time, they could see what was happening and could now understand why I felt the way I did.

The vomiting had steadily increased and we were now at the point where nothing at all was staying down. It was decided that it would be kinder and in Rikki's best interest to stop feeding her. Those last 11 days are my most painful yet precious memories.

We took Rikki into our bed where Joe, who had taken the time off work to be with her and myself, hardly left her side. The girls and Rikki's new carer moved in as well. None of us wanted to miss a single minute with her.

Lots of family and friends came to visit and we tried our best to make those days happy and cheerful....playing her favourite music and singing along. Odd as it may sound, it was almost a party atmosphere at times throughout those days.

I imagine that if you saw us you'd have thought what the hell, but those who were around said it was a privilege to see how happy Rik could still be during such a sad and tragic time. We tried to make her last days as pleasant as we could and show her that if she knew what was happening to her, she had no reason to be scared. I don't think she was.

She even managed to say goodbye by putting her arms out to everyone for cuddles, and that was no easy task for her. It was just like our Rik to be happy, smiling and loving. It was her nature.

On a better note to leave this.... HD hasn't been all bad or sad. We learned a lot of valuable things over the years. Things, many people don't learn in a whole life time. We shared a life time of love and made a life time of memories.

Having Rikki in our family was a privilege.

The Eulogy

On 22nd February 2011, exactly seventeen years to the day from when my husband's father died also having suffered from HD, my husband was cremated.

I had previously arranged services for my parents' cremations, and was taken aback at how there is so much scope for the Chinese whisper affect if the eulogy is based on a short conversation. The vicar misheard my explaining my mother and father had been married for "over forty years". He went on to say "married for forty years" during the Service and, in the process, accidently suggested to all there that my oldest brother had been born out of wedlock!

With that in mind, and with wanting to ensure those around were not given a lecture on the greatness of God, given HD is hardly the best advertisement for all men having been created in God's image (more the Devil's!), I decided to write the eulogy to be read by the chosen 'Life Celebrant'.

As mentioned in the Introduction to Section 8 some of the names have been removed. It probably wouldn't take a degree in genealogy for someone to work out the names of relations given I have put in so much detail alongside our own names but I doubt anyone unaware of HD would just happen upon this book and put two and two together.

I truly hope my siblings-in-law are free from the disease. Being untested at time of writing it is not a certainty. Should the worst case scenario happen I hope what I have done by writing this book will, in some way, go to help them. I just wish more people had shared their experiences and knowledge with me as, until I found the HDA Message Board, even with seeing my father-in-law go through it I can't say I knew anything about caring for someone with such as illness.

In Loving Memory of Steve

We are here today, to celebrate the life of Stephen (Steve) Paul Dainton.

Steve was born in May 1961. The son of Alan and Julia; eldest of 3 children and brother to [names removed]. Husband of Trish.

Steve was academically bright and a natural singer. He was in a church choir and was even in Songs of Praise on the telly. Although Steve joined a church choir, he was not particularly religious. Part of the attraction of joining the choir was he loved being part of an innocent gang with a perceived, guilty pleasure.

He would sneak off with like-minded spirits and listen to Rock music on one of the other boys' tape recorders. Hangman became more interesting. It was clever to know of 'Lynard Skynard' with its use of one vowel when your classmates were still into The Osmonds.

Steve's love of Rock Music, especially the band Queen, remained with him throughout his life. He saw them in concert in the days of Freddie Mercury. He was due to see We Will Rock You again this year for his 50th birthday, having seen the show 6 times already, but sadly it was not to be. Instead, he chose this time to opt for a personal meeting with Freddie Mercury himself in Heaven.

Steve became a Civil Servant in 1978 where he first met a group of friends who introduced him to a great social life and also to his wife to be – Trish. Well... as Trish says "You win some you lose some".

Steve and Trish started dating in August 1987. At the end of February 1988 they were engaged. I'm told by Trish that was due to a bet with a friend and something to do with it being a Leap Year. Apparently this bet backfired according to Trish.

Several months later, Trish finally plucked up the courage to meet her proposed in-laws. Steve later relayed she had looked like a rabbit caught in the headlights half the time. It couldn't have gone too badly though, because they were married in the November of that year.

In November 1988 they married at Wandsworth Registry Office. Rumour has it that the venue was chosen not for its character, but because it was the only place with suitable steps Trish could stand on, so as not to have only the very top of her head in all the wedding pictures.

The height difference didn't seem to matter though... Steve wore a beautiful beaming smile throughout the wedding day and his married life. His smiles were always so full and genuine. Even when later it became harder to physically smile, with his face muscles becoming weaker; and where a lesser man would have given up and felt self pity, he would still try to smile and laugh show his love of life.

Upon marrying, Steve and Trish lived with her mother for a while in Battersea. It was during this period that Steve became a black belt Yahtzee player, such was her mother's love of coercing the poor man into playing board games. He never grumbled, and would always humour his mother-in-law by playing and letting her win. His mother-in-law's love of cooking roast dinners also meant that the black belts kept on needing to be loosened!

After they moved out to buy their own place in Erith, Steve and Trish settled down to a life of work, rest and play. They went on numerous holidays including a luxury cruise arriving in Southampton in style on the Orient Express, flying back on Concorde.

More holidays and cruising followed. Even when Steve's balance was faltering they didn't let it beat them, simply adapting to their circumstances to take a more sedate pace.

They became very fond of Llandudno and Steve achieved his ambition to climb Mount Snowdon, albeit with the aid of a steam train and a can of lager served by the on-board mini buffet for sustenance.

Changes in accommodation to make life easier ensued. He amused Trish when saying at first he felt they couldn't move into the two bed flat they had in Greenwich. This was because there would be no room for his records! But move they did, and the last four years together were spent in Greenwich.

Steve was very aware he was at risk of inheriting Huntington's disease - HD. He would have also been acutely aware of how it affects sufferers...HD having affected his father, and many other relatives. In fact, it was on this very day 17 years ago that Steve lost his father, Alan, to HD. It is fitting that both men died in their lounges, in their chairs with their wives present. Like father, like son. Alan too is in our thoughts and prayers today.

There can be no denying it is never easy dealing with having HD in your life. Steve would get frustrated, agitated and anxious as would anybody in those circumstances. However, his underlying gentle temperament meant that there was never a question mark over his ability to work with Trish in keeping them both independent, and in the comfort of their own home.

The fact that so many care and health professionals personally expressed their sorrow, and were hoping to pay their respects in person today, speaks volumes. He touched so many with his fighting spirit and wit, not least of all his concern for Trish often asking her "you alright?"

Trish and Steve never had children. This was by choice. Knowing that Steve was at risk of inheriting HD, they took the tough decision early on in their relationship. It turned out to be the right decision for them they agreed.

They were fortunate enough to share a love of animals, especially cats. In that sense they had a special fondness for the cats that visited them from a neighbour's garden. Fudge and Sooty. When both cats moved home, Steve pined so much Trish needed to find a suitable substitute. This is when Ruby entered their lives.

Ruby is not like other cats...she allowed Steve to stroke and pat her all day if he wanted and he loved Ruby with a vengeance! Trish will never know if he was just humouring her, and had realised from the start that Ruby was actually an amazingly realistic toy cat.

In fact Ruby was one of five where Trish needed to make sure there was always a cat to respond to. "Has Ruby had her prawns?" was often the morning greeting for Trish. Perhaps Steve was, in his own way, ensuring Trish had company when it was time to say goodbye. Ruby is now pining for Steve

On Thursday 27th January, Steve's struggle with HD became too much for him. He was a fighter but needed to rest. Pneumonia was making it harder than ever for him to keep his spirit up.

Although verbal communication was becoming more and more difficult, he never gave up trying until the very end of his life. He was only able to communicate briefly on that last day though. He had been exceptionally quiet and Flavia - his longest serving carer - tried to rally him by asking, as she always did, if Ruby could come home with her. Steve immediately perked up and said "No" as he always did. It made them both smile to have the old Steve back.

He also mouthed his last words "Home, Home" when Trish gently asked "Hospital or Home". She didn't have to say any more than that, they both knew the time was drawing near and he gave her strength to sit quietly with him, holding his hand. He didn't panic, he slipped away peacefully.

Even after Steve's death he seems to have reached out to loved ones. Steve had a wonderful dry sense of humour, he wasn't one to tell jokes but he was incredibly witty.

Whilst going through paperwork needed for the formalities, Trish and her sister – Brenda – came across an envelope. The envelope had been in the box with Steve's papers for years but Trish had never really looked at the contents.

The letter was a write up for a band Steve had played in whilst at school. It was the most hilarious piece of work and it made them both laugh so much. It was exactly what they needed to read to remind them of how much fun Steve was and it took the edge off the sadness of the task. Steve was saying "cheer up you two!"

And then there was the message to Trish in a song…

With Steve being a great lover of Pink Floyd, Trish was going through Pink Floyd track listings for inspiration for this service. She came across a song called 'The Great Gig in The Sky'. That seemed to fit in with Steve and his love of concerts.

Not familiar with that title, Trish put the record on… The song begins with a man's voice talking over the intro music. She then heard the words…

"And I am not frightened of dying, any time will do. I don't mind.

Why should I be frightened of dying? There's no reason for it, you've gotta go sometime"

"I never said I was frightened of dying".

The words seemed to be spoken just for Trish. It was the reassurance she needed. Indeed, Steve had NEVER said he was frightened of dying. He would now be at peace.

I have only captured a tiny, TINY part of Steve, the man and his life.

A man who packed in so much in such a short few years.

He lived with the shadow of HD over his head but never let it stop him living life to the full. In fact, he was holidaying at Sandringham with HRH as his neighbour even as recent as eight weeks ago – Christmas.

They stayed in Park House on Christmas day, opting out of meeting the Royals on her traditional church visit. Aside from the cold weather making it unwise, Steve had already made his disappointment known. He'd thought Trish meant he could meet members of Queen – the band. Upon realising it was the monarchy he turned his nose up! It was the Queen's loss that she didn't get to meet such a remarkable man.

Steve enjoyed following his beloved team, Crystal Palace, right up to the last few days of his life. That is if the words enjoying and Palace go together given their recent performances before he died.

Then again he is probably that extra bit of wind pushing the ball past the opponent's goal keeper now. Just a few days after his death Palace climbed out of the relegation zone.

I think what Steve would have wanted to say to you all now is to take a leaf out of his book and live for the day.

Do not mourn him. He did more in his 50 years than most people would have done in a hundred.

He was loved by everyone who knew him.

He didn't let HD stand in his way, and never felt sorry for himself.

In the end he achieved his desire... to die at home in a comfy chair with Trish reassuring him it was going to be alright.

End of Eulogy

If you have been touched by the plight of those with Huntington's disease, and would like to make a donation to the HDA, their address is given below.

Alternatively, if you would like to make your donation to the HDA in memory of Steve Dainton who inspired this book, you may wish to donate through his Justgiving Page:

www.justgiving.com/StephenDainton

Thank you! xxx

Huntington's Disease Association Head Office
Neurosupport Centre, Norton Street, Liverpool, L3 8LR
Tel: 0151 298 3298
email: info@hda.org.uk

Lightning Source UK Ltd.
Milton Keynes UK
UKOW02f0653201016

285716UK00001B/42/P

9 781908 105097